COVENANT MEDICINE
Being Present When Present

David H. Beyda, MD

COVENANT PRESS

ACKNOWLEDGEMENTS

Ever since I was six years old, I wanted to be a physician. I wanted to take care of children, and children who were the sickest. Living overseas in underprivileged countries due to my father being a US Foreign Service Officer, I wanted to also take care of children in underprivileged countries. I would accomplish all of that, but not without a lot of help from a lot of people: Henry Beyda, my father, who gave me the opportunity to learn about countries and cultures that few children are ever given, and for sending me to schools that would prepare me for my vocation in medicine. To Samuel Gray III, a cardiologist who took me under his wing when I was a beginning medical student and showed me what it meant to have a "covenant" relationship with patients—and no, he was not faith based, but compassionate and caring, bringing the true sense of the word "covenant" to his relationships with patients; to Edmund Pellegrino, MD, who showed me what it means to be a caring healer in its truest sense by being present when present at the bedside; to David Tellez, MD, and Paul Liu, MD, my two partners, who gave me wisdom and insight when it came to prayer and faith at the bedside and who prayed unceasingly for me; to Charlcye, my wife, for her caring and sacrifices while I spent hours and hours at the hospital and in underprivileged countries, for support and encouragement in my writing and for believing in me; to my sons, Justin and Nicholas, for being patient with me as a father who was absent many times and who both showed me unconditional love; to my daughter-in-law, Rebecca, who was a pediatric resident at my hospital and who traveled with me to Africa on a medical mission, where she met my son Nicholas. They got married a year and a half later. She has a gentle presence with patients, a comforting smile, and gives meaning to being "present when present." To Reverend Robert Stanley, who believed in me and taught me what faith is. God has put you all in my life and I'm so grateful for that. To Dr. Jacque Chadwick who served as a silent mentor, showing me how faith can be powerful even when it is silent. And to the children who were and are my patients and to their families: for showing me the light and for making me realize that they are my first and foremost responsibility to care about and to care for. To serve and to be present when present.

TABLE OF CONTENTS

Acknowledgements iii

Prologue   Who's Jeffrey?..vii

Chapter 1   Who Cares?...1

Chapter 2   Covenant or Contract 5

Chapter 3   Value Principles 14

Chapter 4   A God in a White Coat.....................................20

Chapter 5   Truth Telling 23

Chapter 6   Baby Nicole and Faith 31

Chapter 7   Faith and Medicine 35

Chapter 8   Prayer at the Bedside......................................49

Chapter 9   Covenant and Prayer 52

Chapter 10   The 5 Questions 55

Chapter 11   Do You Treat the Disease or the Patient? 61

Chapter 12   Is the Relationship between the Physician
                and the Patient a Contract or a Covenant? 64

Chapter 13   Is Your Priority Curing or Caring?...................68

Chapter 14   Casey and Technology.....................................74

Chapter 15   Is the Technology We Use a Necessity
             or a Convenience?...78

Chapter 16   High-tech Companies: Responsibilities..........87

Chapter 17   Covenants and Bob 93

Chapter 18   My Uncle..98

Chapter 19   Doctor Nadas..102

Chapter 20   My Friend...107

Chapter 21   Kari 111

Chapter 22   The Dream 115

Chapter 23   Hope, Dignity, and Respect.........................118

Chapter 24   Mr. Morgan 122

Chapter 25   Cure or Care 126

Chapter 26   Caring or Curing—It is Up to Us to Decide......136

Chapter 27   Second-guessing 139

Chapter 28   We are Who We Are 142

Chapter 29   How It Came to Be......................................146

Chapter 30   Self-reflection...148

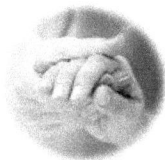

PROLOGUE
WHO'S JEFFREY?

The familiar yet "stop what you're doing" announcement barked loudly overhead. The trauma team was alerted. The trauma team assembled, the high-intensity lights turned on over the gurney, people taking their assigned positions around it waiting to begin the dance of resuscitation with a child who was about to enter. Gowned and gloved, each person silently hoped for the best, but expected the worst. They had all been there before. Many times. The boom of the helicopter's rotors were heard, the team shuffled from side to side, all silent, rehearsing in their minds what they were expected to do. The rotors slowed. All eyes were now turned to the entrance to the trauma bay. Within minutes, a rush of people surrounding a gurney raced through the doors, one person calling out the child's vitals, preliminary assessment of injuries, and a cry for help as they were losing him. The dance began.

He was four years old and not restrained in the vehicle. He arrived in the trauma bay with a severe head injury, multiple fractures, a liver that was bruised, a spleen that was shattered, and more. His face, covered in blood, was pale. A breathing tube was urgently placed down his throat, catheters were threaded into his veins and arteries, limbs were splinted, blood transfused, medicines given to keep his blood pressure up, and he was transferred to the pediatric intensive care unit. We put in more catheters, measuring the oxygenation of his brain cells, put catheters into his brain to measure the pressures that were building up, hooked him up to monitors, and danced a dance of medical interventions that we hoped would make a difference. It was going to be a long night.

❧

"This four-year-old boy arrived last night after being involved in a motor vehicle accident," the resident began. We were starting rounds, I as the attending doctor, and an entourage of residents, medical students, respiratory therapists, nurses, and more. Fifteen people in total. The resident continued with the presentation, citing numbers, results of X-rays, events overnight, and the morning's latest vitals. I took over.

"Cerebral edema is massive, intracranial pressures are uncontrolled, and cerebral metabolism is in jeopardy. The heart is marginalized, liver is failing, the spleen is not functioning, and we have a brain that is ready to burst." I was on a roll with my academic introduction to the physiology of cerebral blood flow, cerebral oxygenation, cardiac output, and more. Taping a large piece of paper to the wall, I began to draw diagrams, figures, formulas, and more. There was rapt attention. The parents were with us, as was customary in our unit. They were encouraged to attend rounds to hear what we said, and to ask questions. We would meet with them again after rounds to go over the care in more detail and to use language that they would better understand.

As I was moving from brain physiology to cardiac physiology, the mother interrupted me.

"Excuse me," she said softly. There was silence. I stopped mid-sentence and looked at her.

"You really don't know who Jeffrey is, do you? All you know is what he is. A bunch of broken pieces that you are trying to put back together." There was more silence. I didn't reply.

"You don't even call him by his name. He is a 'thing' to you. Well, not to me. His name is Jeffrey. He is my son." She turned and walked back into his room. We stood silently for a moment. Each of us had realized how far off the mark we were. Rounds were never the same after that.

Sometimes one needs to get slapped to wake up. And slap me she did and everyone there. We had missed the mark of relationships. We were concentrating on the "what" and not the "who." We talked around the "who" and talked about the "what." It is this very aspect of relationships that I want to share with you. That medicine is centered on a physician-patient relationship based on the "who," the person, and not only on the complaint, the injury, the illness, or the diagnosis. It is about knowing who the patient is, his life, his goals, his wants, and his fears. It is about honesty, integrity, trust, and respect. It is about having a "covenant" relationship between patient and physician. We are used to "contracts," where we hire others to fix what is broken, expecting that all will be fixed and if not, the "contractor" is faulted. Medicine is a lot like that; not all of it, but more and more of it is. I am walking a fine line here implying that there is a disconnect between all physicians and patients. Not so. But as you'll see, it is can be more often than one would expect. I'll tell how we got there and why. I'll give you examples of "contracts" and examples of "covenants." I'll tell the stories that will give you pause to think about your own relationships with patients. I'll talk about faith and how that can bring a physician and patient closer. You may disagree with much that is said, but maybe not. I can only take you there and let you find your own way.

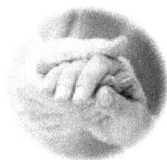

CHAPTER 1
WHO CARES?

*O*n the other hand, who cares? Who cares who Jeffrey is? Aren't we supposed to just get him better and fix him? Isn't that what you want, mom and dad? Isn't that what we want? Isn't that what the insurance company is paying us for and what you expect of us? Is it really important that I know who Jeffrey is? Wouldn't you rather I understand the reasons why his brain is swelling and what I need to do to fix that? Isn't that what we are taught to do ethically? Aren't we supposed to engage the primary virtues in healthcare: trust and beneficence (doing good)? Isn't that supposed to be the end all? To act for the good of the patient, do no harm and to always be clinically competent? Look, if I can get your son home, then won't that be what you want? I can do that. I can keep him alive. So, who cares what his name is?*

❧❧❧

Hard and harsh words aren't they? But, reality begins to sink in when we look at what our society expects of us as physicians: "Cure me and cure me fast. I want the diagnosis now, and the treatment now, and it better work." Well, not all of society I grant you, but I dare say, more than we realize. We find ourselves in a self-centered medium that limits caring for others. I say this not to downplay all those wonderful people who give to others, the servants of society like hospice workers, nurses, social workers, clergy, charitable organizations, and more. You know who you are. You get the point. When push comes to shove, we find ourselves torn between our duty to care for others and our duty to care for ourselves (families included). Do we risk putting our families and ourselves in danger in order to help others? Policemen, firefighters and the armed services do. But even they sometimes find themselves questioning how far should they go when they are faced with danger.

It comes down to who cares. Do I care enough about "you" the "who", to do my best, to make sure that as a physician I ask the question "do I try and keep you alive and send you home with whatever morbidity comes of it, or do I ensure that you leave the hospital with a meaningful life as you define it"? I need to know "who" you are to understand your goals and wishes.

∽∞∽

I witnessed something a few years back that made me realize how uncaring some can be. I was a far distance from the event and when it was over, a policeman gave me the details of "who" this person was. He had known him, seeing him during his beat for several years. The event was not good. Not good at all. For what it's worth it shouldn't have happened, it was unexpected, and it was simply not good.

Somewhere between the sun coming up in the east and the sun going down in the west, Mr. Arrand found himself lost in a city that he had grown up in. At eighty-six years old, he had spent his life as a textile importer in the heart of Manhattan, moving rolls of cloth from the warehouse he owned to clothing manufacturers throughout the States. Having sold his small textile importing business he was retired these past twenty years which had given him time to make up for the years when he never took a vacation, working weekends, and missing out on a family life. Never married, childless, he lived alone from one day to the next working the textiles. During his retirement years he did he same thing everyday. Early to rise, a cup of coffee, a piece of toast and a stroll to Central Park to read the day's paper and to check out the horses running that day at the tract. He never betted. He would check the next day on how he did the day before, and more often than not, he was a winner. If he had been a betting man he would have been living in a posh retirement community in the Florida Keys by now with all the money that he would have won.

But this day would be different. He was in Central Park. Sitting on his usual bench, the paper that he had been reading, now lay at his feet. His face drooped off to the left, his left eye wide open, his tongue protruding off center, drool pooling on his chin and his right arm and leg hung limp, held up only by the fact that he had tilted toward the nylon bag with the worn handles that he bought with him everyday that held a torn windbreaker, a banana and a bottle of water. He looked out towards Central Park, but he didn't see. He couldn't hear. He had had a stroke I would learn later. People passed him, thinking he was a homeless lost person who was sleeping off the effects of alcohol. Three teenagers came up to him, taunted him, and when he did not respond, they pushed him over on the bench and spit on him. And people just walked by. He lay like that for hours until a patrolling police officer came by and told him to move. The police officer turned him over and recognized him. Mr. Arrand didn't respond and an ambulance was called and it all began. All that was to be. All that should not have happened. All that would be with me for a very long time. The people walking by didn't care. The teenagers didn't care. And I wonder just how much the policeman would have cared if he had not recognized Mr. Arrand.

So, who cares?

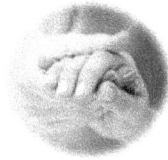

CHAPTER 2
COVENANT OR CONTRACT

Covenants are all about caring. A deep sense of caring. A fundamental difference between a contract and a covenant is that a contract is formed between two persons with written, spoken, or even unspoken agreed upon terms that can be considered binding. A signed informed consent can be such a contract.

The covenant in medicine is different in that it is between a physician and a patient, one who is seeking help and the other offering it. The covenant rests on the concept of servanthood to those who are vulnerable. The covenant brings with it mutual caring: the physician cares about the patient (to do good) and the patient cares about the physician (to trust).

I believe that a contract is built on distrust, hence the legal document, the binding handshake and the consequences of failing to meet the expectations of the contract. A covenant is built on trust. A sincere and honest trust between the physician and the patient, trusting that each will do their best to ensure a good outcome. Even death can be a good outcome if the physician and the patient are honest and prepared. Death with dignity. It is not death itself that causes the greatest discomfort in the relationship, but the dying process. Abandonment, pain, suffering and a loss of dignity. The physician who has a covenant with a patient is there unconditionally from the first day of meeting the patient till the last day. A contract is based on management. A covenant is based on servanthood. A contract lists rules and regulations with consequences if broken. A covenant serves with compassion and grace. A contract is fearful of failure. A covenant is faithful of being there no matter what. A contract operates with the assumption that it can be broken. A covenant operates with the assumption that it is boundless. It puts the other person's needs and interests first.

⚮

The Covenant

There is an old Indian proverb that says when an elephant is in trouble even a frog will kick him. Medicine, the art and the science both, seems to be that elephant struggling to get up. Malpractice suits, lack of trust from patients, physicians who are pressed hard to see more and more patients, patients no longer called "patients" but "customers" or "clients," and health care for those who can afford it, and aspirin for those who can't. But there is hope for recovery. We are all a little older, and a little wiser. They say that what is done is done, that yesterday is yesterday, and that the past is the past. Well, I'm not so sure. The past does come back if only to remind us of what once was and how maybe, just maybe, we can learn from the past and bring forward all that was good and true. No need to reinvent the wheel now is there?

∽◇∽

Every once in a while life intrudes on this love affair I have with medicine. A while back I flew my plane to clear my head and realized how powerful it is to direct and control where one is going and how high one can go. There is always a little turbulence, a couple of clouds that obscure our forward vision at times, but we can climb if we really want to. And I want to climb higher and see medicine for what it was and what it should be. I sense that a cohesive value set in medicine has somehow gotten lost, misplaced, or even unintentionally pushed aside to make room for something else that seems more important. It is that very simple principle of shared values between all who work in medicine that needs to be like a long lost pair of gloves that finally turns up, fitting as well as they did before they were lost.

Have you ever wondered why it is that we have the best of intentions to care for others only to find ourselves doing what we feel most comfortable with: taking care of ourselves? This focus, this time away from caring for others, is what makes us at times self-serving and insensitive to the needs of others. This is not to say that we are always like that, but with time constraints and trying to see a large number of patients in a short period of time, paperwork, insurance forms, billing, etc., we find that our priorities are at times just trying to get through the day without burning ourselves out. There is much talk these days about "self-care". In order to take care of others, we need to take care of ourselves first. I agree. It is how we take care of ourselves that remains the center of the discussions. Is it shortening our work hours? Is it being with family and friends? Is it exercise, hobbies, or something else? I suggest that the covenant relationship I am talking about having with patients, is the same covenant relationship we need to have with ourselves: trusting ourselves to find the best way to stay focused, centered, humble and feeling open to those who care about us.

So here it is. The "covenant." By focusing on establishing a "covenant" with our patients, we can find that we are less prone to be short with them, more honest with them, feel comfortable in conversation with them, and most of all, have a mutual respect for each other's values. This "covenant" brings to the bedside an opportunity to be more than just "doctor and patient." It gives the relationship value and meaning. But with the "covenant" come mutual responsibilities and accountabilities. We hold in trust the interest of each other and we balance our medical expertise with the patients' values.

When I think about a covenant relationship I think about four areas: Action, Listening and Speaking, Intentionality, and Commitment.

Action: How will we change and improve our relationships with patients? We need to balance practical knowledge with wisdom. How can we make the best use of our time and stay a while with our patients? We need understand that we have ownership in this relationship and that we need to work out conflicts and not be shy about it. We need to give assurances and avoid false hopes. We need to remember that for every drug we prescribe, for every treatment we start, we own it. For better or worse. Our actions hold consequences and we are responsible for them. We can't walk away from them. The patient whom we spent days resuscitating only to have that patient survive with a severe disability, is ours. A challenge I give to my partners, residents and medical students, is to go visit the patient three months after they've been discharged out of the intensive care unit and who is now in a long term care facility existing with significant brain injury. Go and see what the consequences were of working hard to just keep that patient alive and perhaps not prioritizing the assurance that they would have a meaningful life once they got discharged. Goals of care, getting to know who the patient is, and what is a meaningful life to them, all give us the information we need to make the hard decisions with our patients.

Listening and speaking: How should we listen to our patients? Silently. We need to be present when present. No multitasking because it compromises the relationship. We speak the truth and do it with grace. We need to share insights and convictions with each other, share personal values, but always remembering that our (the physician's) personal values should never interfere with those of the patient's. Knowing the patient's values is very different than interpreting or guessing what the patient's values and wishes are. As physicians we need to understand that a patient's description of what they believe their quality of life is different that the value of life. That notion needs to be explored by both the patient and the physician. How we define quality and value plays into understanding the patient's goal, wishes and personal values. Simply put, at all times protect the dignity of the patient.

Intentionality: How should we act? Do we make time, do we focus, how do we prioritize, do we do it purposefully and willingly? How do we make the decisions that will affect our patients? Consider that our decisions for treatment should not only be to improve the organs, but it must also be beneficial to the whole patient. We need to be intentional with our patients' trust: we need to balance our medical expertise with the patient's values.

Commitment: What must we give willingly? Always consider the other person's well-being and interests. Embrace empathy and compassion and give quality time in addition to quantity time. Treat patients as persons with dignity, not as commodities. We need to accept risk and be comfortable with self-effacement. Our commitment is to be always centered on the patient preferences. We should treat the patient and never do more to simply increase our revenue. Relative value units (a physician's documentation of service for a fee) inhibit the formation of a physician-patient relationship. We are now seeing reimbursement based on physician performance, where clinical standards are driven by outside sources rather than a physician's knowledge, expertise and experience. This causes a conflict between physician as "gatekeeper" of insurance dollars and being a patient's advocate.

We need to understand that high-tech medicine can threaten relationships and cause conflicts. We need to realize that the events that touch us the most are the ones that we have a covenant relationship with. We need to recognize that with our high-tech society, which embraces contracts, we are left with a lack of a face-to-face community. And we need to understand relationships don't happen by accident. They happen for a purpose.

I believe that we need to fix things, make things right, move forward, and steer straight again. It's the stories that move me, the encounters with those whom I come to help, the ill who look for a better life. I live it every day, here in the United States and in the countries I travel to. And I am more often than not encouraged.

The other day we had a little bit of sadness in the pediatric intensive care unit. A young baby, illness untreatable, came off life support, and what struck me was the intense love of humanism, the unquestioning respect for the dignity of the child, and the selfless acts of genuine caring for that child and each other that was shown and acted on without prompting or protocol. It just happened. Nurses, physicians, respiratory therapists, social workers, and all who came to care about this child. I watched and listened. There was silence and I smiled. There was no need for words, just actions. Everybody got it. Shared values and commitment. A family of dedicated unpretentious people, doing what comes from the gifts that they have been given. When we do what we believe in, serving others in need, unselfishly and together, the sad times hurt less and the joyous times are more joyous.

It is times like those that give me hope that all will be good in the care of patients. For me, it is all about the faith I have in someone more powerful than me, who guides us and asks us to trust Him. This "covenant" that I have with Him is the same covenant that I seek to have with my patients. And for those that are turned off by faith, no worries there. This "covenant" I speak of is universal—a covenant based on an unspoken language of trust, honesty, integrity, and dignity for each other. For both the physician and the patient. So let's climb, gain altitude, look down, and see what we need to see. It's really very nice down there. If we want it to be.

Covenant Diagram

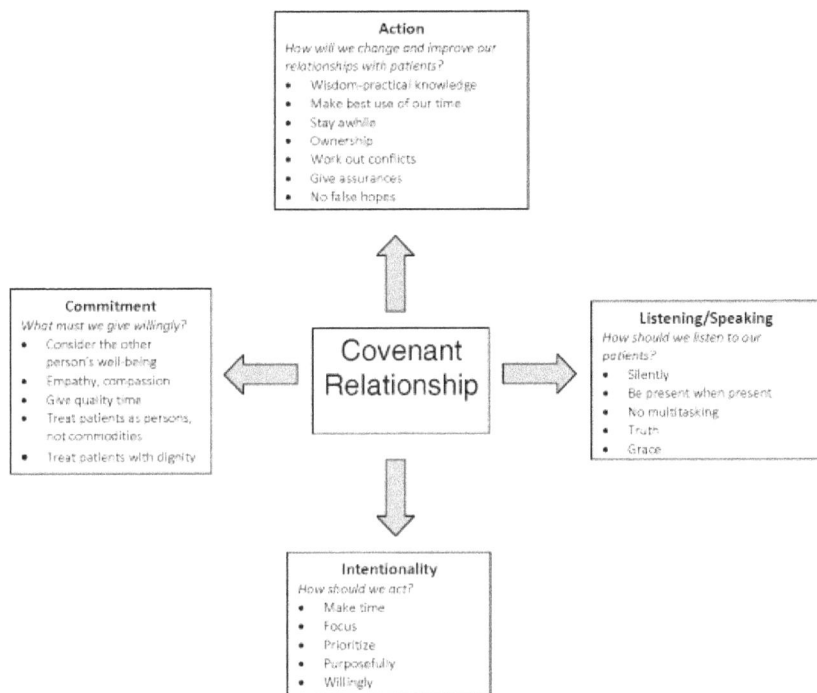

Action

How will we change and improve our relationships with patients?

- Wisdom-practical knowledge
- Make best use of our time
- Stay awhile
- Ownership
- Work out conflicts
- Give assurances
- No false hopes

Commitment

What must we give willingly?

- Consider the other person's well-being
- Empathy, compassion
- Give quality time
- Treat patients as persons, not commodities
- Treat patients with dignity

Covenant Relationship

Listening/Speaking

How should we listen to our patients?

- Silently
- Be present when present
- No multitasking
- Truth
- Grace

Intentionality

How should we act?

- Make time
- Focus
- Prioritize
- Purposefully
- Willingly

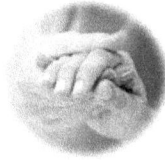

CHAPTER 3
VALUE PRINCIPLES

Medicine's art lies in the sound formation of a relationship between physician and patient. The greatest task physicians have to face is to decide who they are and what their relationship with their patient is going to be. Unfortunately, many physicians' reputations are dependent on how well they cure rather than how well they care. Curing seems to be their only measure of success. Caring is becoming a lost entity in the vocation of medicine, and young physicians today may find themselves unable to care because role models give them the sense that caring is not important. Caring has always been the foundation of medicine. I argue that a physician cannot cure without caring enough to want to cure. Curing and caring are linked and inseparable. Physicians need to refocus their intent to practice caring medicine. In order to do so, physicians must look at who they are. I propose that by asking candid, direct questions of ourselves, we will begin to realize who we are and then either accept who we are or begin to change.

Differentiating between curing and caring can be

argumentative indeed. In order to put them into perspective, I will address each one, defining them as I see them. No pretense is made that both curing and caring are interchangeable. They both are unique, but each works in harmony with the other.

To *cure* implies to make better. It can be very objective and without emotion. A patient is sick and now he is cured. A relatively easy task to accomplish in most cases. To *care*, however, implies a much more personal involvement by both the physician and the patient.

Perhaps there is another way of looking at what caring is. I propose that caring is based on "value principles" individually selected and practiced according to the personality and character of the physician. Physicians can't be everything and all things to all patients. The physician must select those value principles that best suit the needs of the patient with the assumption that a basic foundation of caring principles is held for every patient.

The physician needs a set of "unique values" that can be selected and used. These are what I call "value principles." Each principle produces a different kind of value. A *value principle* must be part of an individual's moral foundation. A *value principle* is a central act that shapes every subsequent plan and decision a physician makes. It therefore defines what physicians do and therefore who they are. Physicians are responsible for all their actions regardless of their intent or lack thereof. My concept of *value principles* forces the physician to make some hard choices and to approach the patient in an honest manner, up-front, without pretense. Caring is a personal matter, biased by a relationship that may or may not be wanting or willingly entered into.

Value principles identify the *caring healer* versus the *curing, health-care provider*. Both types are acceptable, but most patients would prefer the former. The patient must be able to be a partner to the caring healer in order for the relationship to work. Behavior on the part of both the physician and the patient will dictate the type of care given and received. The culture from which the patient comes from and from where the physician comes from will also dictate the type of care given. Value principles come from asking some key questions.

❧

The *value principles* I believe are:

- **Relationship**
  - What type of relationship will you have with your patient: contract or covenant? Will the contract be a commercial or technical one? Will the contract imply success as all contracts do? Will the covenant imply simply a mutual trust, respect, integrity, and honesty between the patient and the physician?
- **Personal commitment**
  - A commitment to do what you *should* be doing or just what you *want* to be doing?

- **Priority**
  - Priority in addressing the needs of cure (disease) or care (patient) or a balancing of both.
- **Technology use**
  - Technology used as a primary resource or as an adjunct.

The following table puts four categories of clinicians into perspective based on a combination of their "value principles":

Value Principles	Curing Health Care Provider	Curing Healer	Caring Health Care Provider	Caring Healer
Relationship	Contract	Covenant	Contract	Covenant
Commitment	Want	Should	Want	Should
Priority	Disease	Patient	Disease	Patient
Technology use	Primary	Primary	Primary	Adjunct

In trying to solve the patient's medical problems, physicians turn to the things they do best. They play from strength, that of their character and principles. The combination of value principles leads to a particular character of caring:

Curing healthcare provider:

The physician rejects traditional medicine and has a tendency to be concrete, formalistic, and sterile in form. He strives for quantification and promotes wholeness of body through science and technology. The curing health-care provider is dedicated to his job, committed to making his patients better in the name of science. He is not, however, willing to take the time necessary to get to know his patients other than in the medical sense. There is no pretense on his part to go beyond the science of curing. A contract is the norm, a business relationship the format. The patient is ill and is seeking help. The physician offers his assistance. A contract is formed, with the buying of services that by virtue of the contract implies a successful outcome. A contract by default would not imply otherwise. No one would enter into a contract if there were a possibility of failure.

Curing healer:

This physician has an empirical approach, devising new methods, new technologies, and seeking new explanations for illness and disease processes. He has a concern for theory and for the most part is a futurist, with a sense of empathy about him. He has an interest in alternative forms of medicine and is curious about their scientific merit.

Caring healthcare provider:

This physician is contemporary and a professional in its purest sense. He has knowledge based on interactions and is driven by such. He is academic and requires scientific evidence of benefit before he uses a particular therapy. He is caring, but at times uncomfortable with it. Science and technology takes precedence over caring.

Caring healer:

This physician ensures patient comfort and dignity by

emphasizing the quality values of life including both the specific and the particular. He is a "classical" physician in the purest sense of the term and promotes wholeness of being.

The caring healer is much more personal in his approach to the patient. A contract is not the guide to the relationship. Rather, it is one based on a patient who seeks help and a physician who is offering it. The relationship is built on trust, integrity, honesty, and respect. No success is guaranteed, although both the patient and the physician will do their best in partnership to bring success about. If the illness persists, there is no blame or fault. An honest assessment is made of the outcome by both the patient and the physician and a decision is made.

Value principles can therefore identify the characteristics of the physician. All four types of physicians may be acceptable, but most patients, I believe, would prefer the *caring healer*. The patient must be able to be a partner to the caring healer in order for the relationship to work. Behavior on the part of both the physician and the patient will dictate the type of care given and received. The culture from which the patient and the physician come from will also dictate the type of care given. We agree to do what we ought to do, not just what we can do.

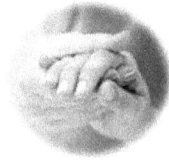

CHAPTER 4
A GOD IN A WHITE COAT

The sky opened up, spilling snowflakes that stuck to each other and all that they touched. The land became covered in a white blanket, but with hidden danger under the soft layer of nature's down. The altitude lent itself to a mark in the landscape that gave this small city a place in the land of retreats from the desert that lay below its suburbs. Flagstaff, at 7,000 feet, rose above the barren land filled with cactus and rock. Flagstaff was a haven from the heat in the summer and a dangerous trek at times in the middle of the winter. The snowfall this time would bring with it an event that would change several lives.

She left Flagstaff late at night, her four-year-old buckled in his car seat in the back on the passenger side. Her husband reminded her to drive carefully. The snow had been falling for some time now, covering the roads with its beauty and its danger. She had driven this highway to Phoenix many times, and knew the places that needed undivided attention and where she could relax and let the road take her where it went. No need for chains just yet. The road was slippery in places, but she had been here before and she was comfortable with it all. Somewhere between the first few miles out of Flagstaff and the beginning of the first descent into the desert, she noticed in her rearview mirror that her son had managed to unbuckle himself and was trying to get out of his seat. She leaned back with her right arm to try and secure him, and lost control of her car. She hit the guardrail, swerved back into the left-hand lane, got hit by a passing car and then thrown over the guardrail, tumbling several hundred feet down the side of a mountain. The little boy was ejected and sustained severe head injuries. The mother was still buckled in when the SUV came to a stop, landing on its wheels. She was conscious when the paramedics got there and refused medical care even though she may have had serious injuries. She pushed away from the paramedics scrambling and looking for her son. She saw him being attended to by paramedics several hundred feet away. They were working quickly to stabilize him and get him to the hospital. They held the mother back, and within what seemed like an eternity, loaded him into a helicopter after they carried him up the steep slope. The mother rode with him and the team in the helicopter, crying and screaming for her son to hear her.

I cared for him when he arrived at the hospital. There was nothing for me to do other than to keep him comfortable. His skull had been crushed and broken like an egg. His mother screamed for me to do something. As compassionate and softly as I could, I told her that there was nothing for me to do.

She began to strike me in the chest with her fists. I didn't try to stop her and simply tried to hold her. Abruptly she stopped, looked at me, and asked, "Are you a Christian?" I said no. She quietly said that God would decide. She slowly turned away from me and climbed into bed with her son and wept as he died. I stood there, arms folded, at first angry at the question, then curious about what she had said about God deciding. I had already decided. I was that "God." A god in a white coat. That was a very long time ago.

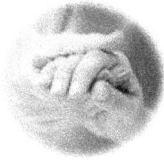

CHAPTER 5
TRUTH TELLING

Some are just incapable of telling the truth and therein lies the problem. Truth has become relative. Social grace allows us to slant the truth just a bit to maintain relationships and to avoid confrontation. So for example, when we see someone, we ask, "How are you?" and the answer is always "Fine, and you?" But it doesn't have to be that way. What if we told the truth? "How are you?" you ask your friend. "Terrible, lousy day, things aren't just right," he says. You stop, thinking, *great, now I've got to stop and listen to this. I should've kept on going*. Try it sometime. Tell the truth to someone who just asked you how you are doing. Say it truthfully and see what happens. Being present when present means being there at all times, for all that is good and bad, and to listen and not only hear.

The lies hit us hardest when we most want to believe them. I have asked the question, as physicians, what is it we are charged to do? Are we curing our patients or caring for them? I think that the real question isn't "what" we do; it's how we do it. Truth telling. Always? Not necessarily.

The day was not starting out very well. Dr. Clemenson was looking over Mr. Simone's labs and the night-shift flow sheet and it boded bad news. A hemoglobin of 6.7, WBC 54,000 with 60 bands, amylase and lipase too high to measure, albumin 0.8, and no urine output all night despite two normal saline boluses. The second patient to be seen on early morning rounds. A lot of time was going to be needed to spend with Mr. Simone this morning, time Dr. Clemenson didn't have. He could come back later, or he could deal with it now. He'd deal with it now. Got a problem, solve the problem. His mind was wide awake, not racing, but just powering steadily along with that special early morning intensity you get in the absence of any other distractions. He got up from the computer and prepared his remarks in his head as he walked to Mr. Simone's room.

Mr. Simone was 68 years old, a blue-collar worker. He was a man of interests and enthusiasms, full of affections and loyalties with middlebrow tastes. He was short and solid and had the kind of worn look a guy gets when he has been in the same line of work too long. He had recently retired from his job as a heavy equipment operator after 50 years. He couldn't remember when he had last taken a true vacation. He was celebrating his 50th wedding anniversary this year, and with the retirement and the wedding anniversary, a real vacation was in order. He and his wife had been set to go on a month cruise around the Hawaiian Islands. Three weeks before they were to leave, Mr. Simone came to see Dr. Clemenson because of a nagging pain in his stomach. He wanted to make sure that he could enjoy the food and the cruise, so he looked to the good doctor for some help. Perhaps a prescription for a powerful antacid for what he thought was an ulcer. It had been there for about two months, off and on. Tolerable, but annoying. Dr. Clemenson found evidence otherwise. An examination and initial labs showed pancreatic involvement and a CT scan confirmed it: pancreatic cancer. Game over. With one week to go before the cruise, Dr. Clemenson sat Mr. Simone and his wife down to "deliver the bad news." He had taken the course on how to do that. Deliver the news factually, softly, gently, honestly, and slowly, he was told. He used to walk in and just tell them. He thought that was the nature of a message—full of tact and rough sympathy, large and intrusive in the neat quiet dwellings of his office or the hospital room, establishing the facts, discussing the outcomes, the therapies or lack thereof, and moving on to the next thing, not caring how or where or why these things happened. He was not in control of them. No use fretting about what you can't control. He had learned to hope for the best, plan for the worst, and facts were to be faced, not fought. Physicians investigate, prepare, and execute. He did all that on the day he met with Mr. Simone and his wife. He told it like it was, delivering bad news the way he had been taught and learned. He told the truth, but his face and his demeanor had already announced it in advance.

They were crushed, canceled the cruise, and Mr. Simone stayed in the hospital for further tests and whatever therapy Dr. Clemenson could muster that would make life more comfortable for whatever short time was left. What Dr. Clemenson was not going to let happen were the aggressive interventions that technology could afford. Technology had already replaced humans in any number of areas, leading to a self-serve economy in everything from grocery store self serve checkouts to ATM banking. But while the technology can allow the temporary illusion of independent self-sufficiency even in medicine (insulin pumps, pacemakers, even ICU monitors), there is something lost in the illusion and cultural self-sufficiency. We lose a richness of tapestry and experience that comes with human contact, a feeling of being a tangible part of a community that works together to make sure all of its members are okay and find their way through the night without harm. The human contact in medicine of having a physician come into the patient's room and sit on the side of the bed and talk. A nurse who comes in and feels a patient's pulse rather than placing an infrared probe on a finger. Mr. Simone was going to get cared about and cared for, not just taken care of. And now after two weeks in the hospital, things were coming to an end.

Several days later in the early morning, Dr. Clemenson got up from the computer and walked slowly to Mr. Simone's room. It was quiet at this time of the morning in the hospital, lights still dimmed, the night staff finishing up their chores, and the sun just beginning to show a ray or two over the horizon. He arrived at the door, took a breath, knocked, and opened it. Mr. Simone was sitting up in bed waiting for him. Dr. Clemenson saw that what was once a fit man was now a man a pale, thin, and drawn shell of a man on the way down the wrong side of the hill. A man yielding gracefully to the passage of time without getting all stirred up about it. And yet he also saw the dull mist of worry hanging just in front of his eyes. The lines between hope and despair. It was about helplessness, submission, and powerlessness. It is said that those who are terminally ill contemplate death every waking moment and even when asleep. Some live with it, some expect it. Most eventually accept it. Some of them even want it. But deep down they want it to be fair. They want it to be noble. Win or lose, they want it to arrive with dignity.

"'Morning, doc. How's life?" Mr. Simone said, his voice now hoarse with dryness from failing kidneys.

"So far so good, Mr. Simone. The sun's coming up, the world is waking up, and I get to see you first on my list of patients."

"So how am I doing?" said Mr. Simone, a faint smile on his cracked lips.

Dr. Clemenson was about to answer when his mind journeyed back a few years to an old mentor who had given him advice that was now stored in the recess of his memory bank, brought out from time to time when the need was there. There was need now. Was his mentor always right? No. But that extra piece of wisdom, gleaned from years of experience and patient care, gave him another valuable piece of information to put into his decision-making equation. This was far from the only time he'd gained tremendously from heeding the wisdom of an experienced physician, but this time, he was going to move into an area of ethical danger. Lying. He was about to embark on a path that some find rocky, and others would not even tread. But why? We lie all the time. It is the most common act we do, every day, many times over, without even knowing we do it. It is habitual in character and nature. We do so because it is socially accepted. It's called "tact" or "social grace." Lying avoids conflict, prevents discomfort and disruption, until it is found out. Then we're in trouble. But what if the party to whom we are lying in fact wants us to lie? Does that make it right? For Dr. Clemenson, this truth telling as a moral obligation ran deep. Veracity or telling the truth was a virtue that had always run parallel to his life. And in medicine, the truth should trump all. So they say. But it's how you tell the truth that matters. And why you tell the truth. To give an honest perspective to what the patient has in store for them. They need to know. They need to look forward, not backward. They need to concentrate on what's ahead. It is what they need to hear, because it is true. They need a story. An explanation. The who, the where, and the why. Every patient needs to know what is happening to him or her and what is going to happen. But here's the rub. Even when we tell the truth, people, patients, see and hear what they want to see and hear. It's how they cope. It's what they feel comfortable with. Truth or not.

There are times when the truth is not the best answer and a variant of the truth is. Ethics dictates that we do what is best for our patients. Not always right, but best. Doing what is good for the patient, the humanistic side of medicine, a pervasive concern for human welfare. And kindness. Kindness counts for a lot, and is a factor in medicine that brings with it the touch of the physician-patient relationship that both patients and physicians look for. Kindness can sometimes make us lie, especially when our patients are walking in a dead man's shoes. We lie to our patients out of kindness; it is a virtue that runs parallel to our vocation of service. It's what our patients may need to hear, even when it is a lie.

"Hey, doc! You with me? How am I doing?" Mr. Simone said, pulling Dr. Clemenson back to time and place.

Dr. Clemenson rose out of his deep recess of thought and looked over at Mr. Simone. He walked over to a chair, pulled it close to Mr. Simone, and took his hand.

"You're going to be fine, Mr. Simone. Just fine."

Dr. Clemenson said what he needed to say, and Mr. Simone heard what he wanted and needed to hear. That he was not alone and that he would be cared about. Dr. Clemenson could have easily said, "Your blood counts are very concerning and getting worse, your kidneys are failing, and I think it's just a matter of time." The truth. But he didn't. He said Mr. Simone would be fine. Not cured, no change in outcome, but fine. Implied comfort, pain free, and dignified. Was that a lie? A variant of the truth? A mixed message? Some would think so. False hope? Lying or withholding the truth to give hope in a situation where there really is none is not right either. But there was no mention of a cure or change in prognosis. Did Mr. Simone need to hear the details of his impending death? Dr. Clemenson didn't really think so. He believed that honesty is a virtue; therefore lying is bad except when perhaps telling a lie is a result of another set of virtues: compassion and kindness. And perhaps compassion and kindness trumps all. Even telling the truth.

Mr. Simone smiled and held Dr. Clemenson' s hand for a very long time. A strand of melancholy that was there before gave way to the afterglow of two people coming together, one seeking help, the other giving it, without pretense or expectations. Just silent understanding that what is, is, and that there is room for already knowing the truth without it having to be told.

A person less fortunate than ourselves deserves the best we can give. Truth be told, Dr. Clemenson gave it his best and Mr. Simone deserved no less.

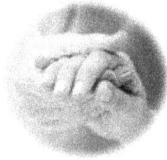

CHAPTER 6
BABY NICOLE AND FAITH

The alarms were going off. Heart rate 60, blood pressure falling. The persistent chiming of the harsh, abrasive chirp gave warning to an end of a life. Standing by the open warmer, I looked down at the baby, pale with a hue that now was turning blue, and paused for just a second as I battled with my inner thoughts. Push on or accept the inevitable? Out of the corner of my eye, I saw the family sitting close together watching my every move, drawn faces, eyes hollowed by nights of lack of sleep, and expressions of fear and pleading. Two nurses at my side were waiting for orders, for directions to intervene, anticipating what they thought was going to happen next, yet still not sure if it was the right and best thing to do. It had been a long battle. I began chest compressions, called for resuscitation medications, closed my eyes for a brief second if only to seek out some internal guidance that might be buried somewhere in the recesses of my mind, found none, and so took up arms to accept the fight. The alarms kept going. I was going to have to surrender.

Something was about to happen and I was not going to be able to change it. The phone call came late one evening, a woman's voice on the other end, frantic, almost pleading, telling me who she was and why she was calling. I was not on call that night, one of the few nights that I was fortunate enough to have off as a pediatric critical care physician. My specialty was caring for the sickest children, those who required intensive care, who had been critically injured, or who had a critical illness. My training was to try and save the lives of children who were trying to die, and for the most part I was successful. There were times when I lost the battle, but I never gave up. I knew the woman. She was the wife of the senior pastor at the church my wife and two sons attended. I would too, on occasion, as a token of "family" unity. My personal relationship with God was far from solid, nor satisfying. It was not close to being a covenant relationship.

"Can you come to the hospital?" she said.

"What's wrong? Which hospital?" I asked, confused as to what the call was about.

She spoke in short sentences, some broken with a tear and some spoken in a whisper.

"Our brand-new little granddaughter is very sick and just got admitted to your intensive care unit. They say she may die."

That got my attention. I told her I'd be right there.

One never knows what to expect when a patient comes in to the intensive care unit other than I know I'm up for a battle against a body that is in a state of disorder, and I have to try and make it right again. And that is exactly what I faced when I walked into the unit and saw a one-week-old baby girl, pale, weak, and already on life support with doctors and nurses surrounding her, each playing a specific role, each trying to make order of the chaos that encased this little baby's body. Baby Nicole. Born one week ago and headed for an early death.

I spent the next week on a constant twenty-four-hour watch caring for her. That I did these things well was a given; otherwise I would not be in the position that I was. She was attached to monitors, a ventilator, tubes going in her and tubes coming out of her. A rampant infection had invaded her body, taking one organ after another as if they were trophies. I was having a tug-of-war with death, or was it God, He pulling her to Him and me pulling back? I had no intentions of letting this little baby die. It was becoming clear however, that I was not going to win.

During her week in intensive care, I had several discussions with the family and with Rev. Bob Stanley about the possibility that Nicole was going to die. On a Friday morning, I approached the family and shared with them that it was time to take Nicole off of life support. I had reached the end of the rope that held her delicate life, and the rope was becoming threadbare. There was nothing that I could do or could offer.

The medications that I had running through her veins were keeping her alive, and without them she wouldn't survive. Without any question or anger or frustration, the family understood and agreed. I placed baby Nicole in her mother's arms, took the technology away, stopped the medications, and left them alone. As I was stepping out of the door Rev. Stanley called my name. As I turned around, he simply said,

"David, it's all about faith."

I turned and walked out, not really understanding what he meant. If somebody should die, it clearly was Nicole. There was no way she was going to make it with the infection that she had, faith or no faith. I thought about that word "faith" from time to time. I even tried to explore its meaning once, but never got very far. But one day it made sense. I made a journey from being a God in a white coat to a servant, to a physician in service to and for others. I struggled with whether my focus was blurred, or just a little off balance. I learned that it is about faith and prayer and a covenant with my patients. I found how a deepened sense of spirituality could benefit both the physician and the patient. I found what it meant to be virtuous and how that is what and how we are supposed to be.

It's all about faith.

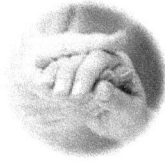

CHAPTER 7
FAITH AND MEDICINE

A conversation was overheard between two children who were visiting their ill grandmother in the hospital. The first asked, "Why is Grandma spending so much time reading the Bible these days?" "I guess she is cramming for her final exams," the second replies. To imply that when science has nothing more to offer it turns to religion is not the message here. It does imply that patients, persons who are sick, are in need of a different type of science, one that goes beyond the rituals of cure. Physicians do well as providers of cure under the guise of science, but some fall short as providers of faith— a spiritual dimension that goes beyond science. What therefore is the proper scope of medicine? Should the scope of medicine be broadened to include spirituality, faith, religion, and prayer? Under what circumstances should medicine give way to the spiritual, religious, and faith needs of the patient? Should the physician use spirituality, faith, and/or religion without the patient's consent? What do spirituality, faith, religion, and/or prayer and scientific medicine have to do with one another? Should they be kept independent? Should one be subordinated to the other? What contribution does or can one make to the other?

I suspect that some physicians, regardless of their beliefs or non-beliefs in a deity, will at some time use spirituality, faith, religion, and/or prayer in their practice of medicine. The scope of medicine is broad, contrary to a notion that medicine today is all pure science because of the heavy use of technology and drugs.

Physicians believe that humans are worth caring for. So do religions. Both the ministry and medicine encompass a "calling" by virtue of its service to humanity. The white coat may be thought of as a sterile barrier, but has in it the connotation of "god"-like. The white coat may be a robe, a uniform of sorts, unique to the profession, unlike that of a priest. We begin to see that the physician has the opportunity to minister despite the fact that to some, the physician's interest in the patient can sometimes be seen as transparent sincerity. Today, a person looking for spiritual help is far more likely to seek a religious representative.

There are four major areas of healing. They are physical healing, spiritual healing, emotional healing, and demonization. Medicine in and of itself seems to address only one aspect of healing, the physical side. Since the human body has the potential to regenerate or renew or restore itself to health under certain favorable conditions, medicine is the medium through which health is restored. There may be in fact two aspects of the patient's health that need attention: the patient as a physical being and the patient's soul, or spiritual nature, which implies the presence of spiritual illness and the need for spiritual healing. The usual connotation of the word "soul" is religious, denoting that aspect of the human, which relates to the divine saved by religious faith and/or practice.

Good doctors evaluate illnesses by questioning and listening and by a careful visual inspection of the body. This quality, the art of listening, allows the patient and the physician to explore issues other than just the patient's illness. We are unfortunately unable to use this quality adequately in today's medical culture. Physicians are seeing an increasing number of patients in shorter amounts of time. Emphasis is on diagnosis and cure: disease first, patient second.

Physicians have the power of medicine at their disposal. What other qualities must they possess? What makes a physician is not a single skill or a set of skills, but a combination of skills, knowledge, and ability. Where do spirituality, faith, and religion come in? Physicians are fallible and vulnerable and I believe that sometimes they require outside help: spirituality, faith, and religion. A balance between cure and healing begins to emerge. The physician as healer should be founded on the appropriate use of science, spirituality, faith, and religion at the bedside.

I believe that the true physician is the one who takes upon himself the responsibility of healing and helping, not as a negotiated task, but as an imperative built into the very nature of clinical medicine. The inequality of power between physician and patient may be simply rectified by using spirituality, faith, and/or religion if both the patient and the physician agree. They impart a sense of common ground upon which the patient and the physician can work together, no different than both the physician and patient wanting to seek wellness.

Medicine directs what we believe the patient is entitled to and what we perceive the care we give the patient to be. From the point of view of the patient, the vulnerable human being is entitled to receive comfort, care, and a respect for dignity. From the point of view of physicians, we are entrusted to deliver care, ensuring the patient's autonomy, comfort, and dignity. Times have changed, however. I take a risk in saying that some physicians have become self-centered in their priorities, considering their own accolades as important.

◦◦◦

What is the role of faith at the bedside and how do we address the particularity of faith as expressed by both patients and physicians?

Faith may simply be a belief in something. I interpret faith as a leap from religion, considering faith as a need or a desire. Faith encompasses doubt and assumes an intuitive or inherent need to rely on something that is unexplainable. Faith is the foundation of any covenant and entails a strong conviction with a capacity to feel. Faith is simply believing in something with no need for proof.

Faith has two components: *intellectual* and *emotional*. The intellectual component looks for the simple, logical answer, knowing that it is elusive but worthy of search. The emotional component involves a level of comfort in not having to know why.

Faith can be manifest by a reliance on a person and God. There have been arguments that faith can simply be explained by a reliance on something: a car has brakes, and we have faith in those brakes to stop the car. I suggest that this simple example does not do justice to faith. I do not have faith in my car brakes. I have expectations. I expect that my brakes will work. Faith holds no expectations. Faith holds true unconditional certitude to a belief.

Faith can be described as an attitude of the entire self, including both will and intellect, directed toward a person, an idea, or a divine being. This total existential character of faith distinguishes it from the popular conception of faith that identifies it with belief as opposed to knowledge.

Physicians have faith in their ability to cure. And when a cure is not possible, they have faith that they can comfort—all physicians.

Is there a difference between the spiritual and the religious? Patients may indicate that they have no spiritual or religious need, when, in fact, the dogma of religion is not wanted but some faith-oriented spirituality is being asked for. Religious care is that which helps people maintain their belief system and worship practices. Spiritual care is that which helps people identify meaning and purpose in their lives and maintain personal relationships and transcend a given moment.

Of all the characteristics religion has associated with it, a belief in a deity holds the most weight when it comes to physician-patient interaction. An agreement on who this deity is of prime importance in beginning to establish a relationship. There are three main philosophical views regarding the existence of a deity. Atheists believe that no deity exists. Theists believe in a deity or deities. Agnostics say that the existence of a deity cannot be proved or disproved. As an aside, deism holds the view that God exists but takes no interest in human affairs. He wound up the world as a clock and then left it to run itself down.

Medicine and spirituality have often been viewed as mutually exclusive domains. In fact, medicine has been interpreted as unfriendly and even hostile to religion and spirituality. But there is a growing interest in the relationship between medicine and religion, and this may be due to a reaction to the increasingly technological and impersonal nature of medicine today. It is clear that patients are more than the sum of their symptoms. Exploring a patient's religious experience may be beneficial in identifying a source of insight into conflicts and a reservoir of untapped strength that could be useful to both clinician and patient.

But could the incorporation of religion or spirituality into treatment be potentially dangerous? The danger lies in exploitation. The vulnerable patient can be exploited at the benefit of the clinician. We need to emphasize the difference between gathering information about a patient's spiritual life and explicitly or implicitly telling patients how to live their lives. At the same time, almost any kind of strong belief system has the potential to become an ideology that is toxic to therapy and harmful to the patient. For some, science becomes the religion and the technology and science itself becomes the comfort for the patient.

Clinicians must become more sensitive to the patient's religious and spiritual needs. Patients are more likely to be significantly influenced by their own religious backgrounds and beliefs when making decisions. So will the physician. The clinician that wishes to be sensitive to a patient's values must have some awareness of the patient's religious beliefs or lack thereof.

Is praying for the sick intended to heal or comfort? Is prayer intended to direct divine health? Why is prayer necessary and whom does it serve? By praying to remedy one problem, do we create or allow another problem to impact the patient? Physicians begin to understand a patient's beliefs not only by honestly earning them in a covenant relationship, but also by stifling their personal doubts. What about unanswered prayer? What would the effect be on a sick person if we prayed for their healing but no improvement was felt? Prayer allows a sense of ultimate belonging. Physicians who pray with their patients transcend the contractual relationship to one of a covenant. Patients expect their physicians to follow a "virtue model." The patient expects the physician to be a virtuous, moral person whose character has been nurtured and trained. At the same time, prayer can be inappropriate because it might erode the images of confidence and authority that may be desirable in the practice of medicine. Nonreligious physicians who hold on to some degree of faith may perhaps pray more often than not. Silent prayers may be self-directed or focused on their patients. It is prayer all the same. Spirituality is personal and is not always something to be advertised. It grows naturally. At the same time, I have great difficulty in accepting that God favors only those who have others praying for them or are praying for themselves. I believe that God also embraces those for whom prayer is not offered or practiced.

Prayer can be all encompassing or it can reach out and touch a particular emotion. Prayer can be a cry out for help. Prayer can be one of praise where, for example, the dying patient is not praying to say "please help me live," but to say "thank you for taking me into your arms." This prayer of praise is a prayer of gratitude. There is a prayer of silence, which is the simple act of union with the deity to whom the prayer is offered. What prayer does for us as physicians and patients is give us a sense of ultimate belonging to God and each other.

⌒⦰⌒

When routines are ritualized, do you need consent? Is ritual being used to delude patients? Ritual is a pervasive form of human conditioning. When prayer becomes a procedure of a public ritual, it may require consent or at least awareness on the part of the patient. What if a surgical team prays before starting every operation and it is standard practice? Let's say the patient is an atheist and finds out later that a prayer was said prior to the incision. The patient may take affront to it. The surgical team has the right to pray for himself or herself and *for* the patient, but perhaps not on *behalf* of the patient without the patient's consent or knowledge. I pray with my patients and often pray for my patients, but do so in the spirit of bringing God directly into the picture. To assume that my prayer speaks on *behalf* of the patient is still a task that I struggle with. Do I really know what that patient is seeking from their God?

Many times prayer on behalf of the patient includes asking that a miracle take place that would restore physical health. It should also ask that the patient be granted the courage and strength to accept the things that have occurred. Is it appropriate to pray with patients? Is it appropriate to pray for patients? Praying for and with patients can relieve spiritual distress. Prayer is an intimate conversation between a person and God.

Should a strong believer of any religion witness to another even if not asked to? Physicians who evangelize are thought to overstep their professional responsibilities. I would agree only if the patient has not requested such a discussion or is put in a compromising position, i.e., feeling coerced into being witnessed to out of fear that the physician will neglect his medical needs. I have no argument with evangelizing at the bedside if the patient has requested it or has sent a message to the physician opening the way for discussion.

I suggest that treading lightly is the best course. A covenant can quickly turn into a conflict.

Physicians who are faith based should carefully examine their mission: to minister or to evangelize. To minister, to simply care, involves a deep sense of faith and spirituality regardless of an association, or lack thereof, to a deity. To evangelize without permission goes beyond the boundaries of medicine and ministry and becomes a religion-based instrument that may disrupt the physician-patient relationship.

Do patients receive the care they need? Do patients need the care they receive? The physician should have complete acceptance of the patient's belief or preferences, however they may conflict with the physician's conscience or professional judgment. The physician must have the capacity to stand faithfully giving support to his or her patient, regardless of the demands it places on them as a person. Support of the patient's religious beliefs goes beyond the period of illness. It is incorporated into a period of dying, and eventually death. Physicians cannot go wrong by introducing the notion of spirituality, faith, and/or religion in the care of patients. Religious beliefs significantly affect how individuals feel about life, death, and health care.

Diagnosis of a severe illness or terminal illness often precipitates an increased sense of existential urgency and spiritual need and the use of religion as a coping strategy. Serious, life-threatening events seem to be appropriate opportunities for religious inquiry. This can be dangerous because of the vulnerability of the patient. There is a need for physicians to consider and respect the religious and spiritual beliefs of patients. Physicians often fail to identify the spiritual needs of their patients, either because of deficient education as to the need, a perceived or real inability to help, or the specific attitudes and beliefs of the individual physician. The use of spirituality and faith at the bedside becomes unspoken mostly because physicians are striving to reach a balance of comfort and care with science and technology.

A great many things have gone wrong with the world that God has made, and He insists on our putting them right again. Practicing medicine without spirituality is one of them. Medicine at times is not neat, not obvious, not what we expect. Disease may be nothing more than an alteration in the normal function of nature. On the other hand, nature, in its natural course, induces hostile environments that people tend to fight with technology: in the winter we use heat, in the summer we use air-conditioning. The fact is, we constantly react to a change in nature by using interventional techniques that may serve no purpose other than to disrupt the natural course of things or to prolong the result. The romantic form of dealing with nature is to do nothing. Leave it alone and appreciate it for what it is worth.

When physicians battle disease, in a sense nature and God, some think it worth the risk to win at all costs, even to the end of saving a vegetative patient. Physicians assume an attitude that their role is to save lives and thus are absolved of the pain and suffering they now have caused. Since they cannot be blamed for the outcome, they perceive their mission as fulfilled. I look at it differently. I strive to distinguish between just keeping a patient alive, and ensuring that when they leave the hospital they have a meaningful life. A meaningful life as they want it. I explore their goals of care, who they are, and who they are looking to be. By asking the hard questions, survival is defined by their "who" and not by their "what." The superior physician, I should like to believe, is always aware of how little he or she knows. Arrogance contributes nothing other than a display of inconsistencies and insecurities. Physicians can be somewhat authoritarian and paternalistic. Patients request autonomy: the moral right to choose and follow one's own plans of life and action. Physicians are supposed to have respect for this autonomy and refrain from interfering with wishes unless they pose a threat to the patient or someone else.

The social commitment of the physician is to prolong life and relieve suffering. Physicians must get to know their patients as individuals, in a sense become one with them if they are to make valid treatment decisions. They must be able to think reflectively about the patient. It is a difficult task to judiciously balance the role of the patient and family input into often difficult medical decisions with the exercise of sound professional judgment. The manner in which people are treated is as important as the drugs and other therapeutic measures that are used. It has been said that it is sometimes difficult to strike a balance between good judgment and experience: good judgment comes from experience, but unfortunately, experience comes most often from poor judgment. Some physicians practice "selective ignorance" or avoid the issues that are so important to the patient.

It can be argued that at some point in a physician's career, a peculiar challenge of being very much alone with a serious problem or task occurs. The apparent dominance of technology and the loss of opportunities for developing personal relationships with patients make the physician choose the easy way out. The biomedical technologies have also served as barriers to religion, faith, and spirituality in the practice of medicine. They are brought to the forefront. At what point does or should spirituality enter into the care of the patient?

A paradox exists which could easily mislead both the physician and the family. When can a physician feel comfortable bringing religion to the patient's bedside? Doing so may leave the impression that the physician is lacking in scientific skills and must resort to prayer to compensate for his deficiencies. Physicians who fight for a patient's life knowing that it will lead to great suffering and pain or survival in a vegetative state are driven by pride. By judiciously balancing spirituality and medicine in the care of the patient, the physician may achieve harmony with his own heart and brain. The role of the spirituality, faith, and religion in medicine therefore may need to be looked at in "balance" with technology. Physicians will use spirituality based on their beliefs or lack of, their realistic expectations of the outcome and their own limitations. So in fact, when used in "balance," there need not be any winner. To avoid God's interaction is to discard the physician's commitment to use all in his power to comfort and care for the patient.

There is and will always be an absolute limit to what physicians can do for their patients. Accepting this fact can be very hard to do. Physicians are not gods. We physicians are not different from anyone else. There are no "gods in white coats." It seems to me that after all is said and done, after all the science, medicine, and technology is used up, the most powerful act we have left to do for our patients is to reach up, stretch, and touch the hand of God and say: "Thy will be done on earth as it is in heaven." God can surprise us once in awhile.

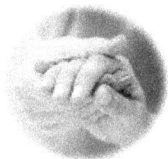

CHAPTER 8
PRAYER AT THE BEDSIDE

In order to establish a covenant with patients, not only must we address the medical and physical sides of an illness, but it is also important that we obtain a spiritual history. A simple question, "Do you have a faith to help you at a time like this?" can be a simple yet exciting entrance into a new dimension of medicine and covenant with a patient. If the answer is no, is a physician obligated to continue looking for an opening to evangelize or should he move on? If the patient answers no to the question of having a faith, would you, or should you, follow up with, "For me, knowing that there is a God who loves us and cares for us is the only thing that makes sense of problems like this." Is that judgmental? Is that burdensome to the patient? Or, is it an opportunity for the patient to reflect on something he or she may not have?

I believe that we cannot go wrong by gently introducing the notion of spirituality, faith, and/or religion in the care of patients. But we must do so with respect for others and for understanding if the patient is not receptive.

There is no monopoly on the part of the physician when

it comes to treating the patient. At the same time, prayer and spirituality may not have a monopoly either. This is evident by the often lack of success of prayer alone in the care of the critically sick patient. It seems that there is a partnership, a common bond and goal in caring for the patient. Spirituality and medicine joined together. There may not be a tug-of-war as such. Physicians don't really pull their patients from the "jaws of death," do they? A "tug-of-war" implies a winner and a loser. If the patient dies, who loses? The physician? The patient? No one would say that God lost. Are we "instruments" of God, directed by some unseen force, some special guidance?

But whatever you believe about prayer and its place in medicine, I believe there is never a better time to thank Him for our blessings and grace than when we see how tiny we are in the great scheme of things...holding the hand of a small one-month-old infant with pus in her eyes, comforting the old man who is trying to catch his breath in between his coughing fits, looking into the eyes of a young women with three young children who tells you she is HIV positive and that she knows she will be dead in a year and she has no one to take care of her children...and could she leave them with us?

⚬⚭⚬

On a trip to Honduras, I saw a Hassidic Jew and his young sons put their tallitot on and pray openly at an airport. Then I met a local pastor in Honduras who had a shofar (a ram's horn) in his church that he blew every Friday before the

Sabbath and blew it for me as he and I recited a classic Jewish prayer. Sitting in the airport in Honduras on the way home, a family of Mennonites was sitting right across from me praying from a book that I didn't recognize.

From all of this, God has been prayed to on many different levels, from different faiths, and perhaps for different reasons. But the fact remains that prayer occurs. He listens better than we do, I suspect, and responds in His own way. A Jew, a Christian, and a Mennonite...how different...how similar.

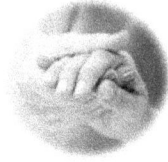

CHAPTER 9
COVENANT AND PRAYER

The attitudes underlying the practice to do "good" for all our patients seem not out of keeping with the spirit of healing that we all subscribe to. But nobody is at his best every day. And that includes those of us who call ourselves physicians. Despite our best intentions, we have on occasion made either small or large errors in our practice. Although medicine is supposed to be a science, there is certainly a great deal of experimentation that takes place, which in itself is prone to error. To think that physicians are far from the common road traveled is to bask in the realm of idealism. Our patients and their families, and yes, some of our own colleagues at times, do not readily accept this very human character that we possess. The feeling that lives are at stake lends credence that error is unacceptable. However, there must be a degree of realism in the approach to the difficult patient. I concede that as a physician I hold no special enchantment, no singular magic.

But what I do know is this. The covenant relationship isn't hard to establish. It doesn't take so much time out of your day that you can't ask a few simple questions and then listen—really listen—to the answers.

Here's an example of what I do. Let's say I have just spent three hours resuscitating that little boy, Jeffrey. He's alive, stable, and it's time to go meet his family. After long exposure to such meetings, I know that they are going to want to know three things: am I qualified, is Jeffrey alive, and what's it going to be like if he survives?

So I walk into the waiting room and I say, "Hello, I'm Dr. Beyda, a critical care physician. I've just spent two hours resuscitating Jeffrey. His heart rate is stable, but I don't know what's going to happen in the next three to four days. That's what we'll talk about. But before we go any further, tell me about..." I then ask them to tell me a little bit about who Jeffrey is, who they are, what their family is like. I wait because I know what's going to happen next. They stop. Their faces change. They see me in a different light as I do them. We're starting to build a relationship of trust.

Once I have that conversation, I tell them, "I'm going to make you three promises: I won't do anything *to* Jeffrey. Everything will be *for* him. He'll always be comfortable and pain free, and I'll always maintain his dignity."

Dignity is of vital importance to humans. No matter who you are or what you have been through, you deserve to be treated with dignity. All parents want this for their child who is in a critical care setting. We all want this as human beings.

Then I tell them, "You and I will be talking frequently over the next hours, the next few days, and I want to be clear that there is a difference between *expectations* and *hope*. I need you to be careful with your expectations, because if they're not met, you set yourself up for failure. If we have hope—--if it works, great, if it doesn't then we know we never gave up." What this final comment does is set the tone for the covenant. If I kept it simply as a contract, then there's an expectation that the child is going to get better. That doesn't always happen in my vocation. But the covenant allows for hope, and yes, at times acceptance of the frailty of life.

I ask them if they have a faith they turn to, both when times are good and when times are less than stellar. If they say yes, we explore that faith, I offer them support from their denomination or their house of faith, and I share with them that I believe in a God, one who is all knowing and a God to all. There are no boundaries when it comes to God. I wait for an appropriate moment to ask them if they would like to pray with me.

It's that quick, and it makes all the difference in the world.

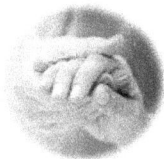

CHAPTER 10
THE 5 QUESTIONS

I bring up the "care" versus "cure" question again to hopefully make you aware of something important. Whether you are a doctor or a patient, you must know that in our current world of insurance-based decisions, what seems to have been pushed aside is the personal aspect of medicine. It is thought to be of no importance. It's not needed. But how could it not be? Recently however, there is a push to grade physicians based on their bedside manner. One can search for "Healthgrades" of physicians and even get comments and recommendations from patients on those "Healthgrades" lists. I wonder if the comments and grades are related to good versus bad outcomes. When patients are cured, the physicians get an "A" grade. When things don't go just right or as the patient wants it to through no fault of the physician, the grade drops dramatically. Seems like it is all "contract" based, doesn't it?

Medicine is about people helping people. We're not gods in white coats. We're men and women trying our level best to help our patients—to either get better or die gracefully. But there is a lot of middle ground in between those stark opposites: the time needed to establish a relationship, the privilege of doing so, the necessity of doing so, and the must of doing so.

To really understand the importance of that middle ground, it is vital that we all ponder and eventually answer the following questions:

1. Are we treating the patient or the disease?
2. Is the technology we use a "necessity" or a "convenience"?
3. Are we doing something "for" the patient or "to" the patient?
4. Do we care or do we cure?
5. Do we have a contract or a covenant with our patients?

If we "care" rather than "cure," if we treat the "patient" (the person) and not the "disease," and if we use technology because it is "necessary" for the patient and not a "convenience" for us (we can attend to other things, personal things, "me" things, rather than being with the patient), then "caring" becomes central in our relationship: it's about "who," not about "what."

Caring is supposed to come naturally, or so it is thought. When I ask myself the above questions, I am honest. Yes, I have often cared enough to visit my patients when they needed comfort. No, I do not visit my patients often enough when all they need is comfort.

The simple truth is, anyone can "take care of" somebody: that's simply mechanics. But to "care about" and to "care for" somebody takes self-sacrifice and an intent to be there for someone regardless. It takes commitment, and that gets to the heart of the matter: having a covenant relationship with our patients. In order to grasp the enormity of the covenant relationship, let me revisit what used to happen, back when physicians and patients lived and worked together in small communities.

About a hundred or two hundred years ago, relationships between physicians and patients were based on shared values. Shared values, those inherent virtues, those characteristics that people look to in others, are what bring relationships together and cement them. Within the community a physician was well known and in turn the physician knew the community members. There was a personal relationship between all of them based on the fact that the communities were small, there were daily activities that everyone shared, and everyone knew each other.

Physicians from long ago would carry with them a black bag, and within that black bag they would have several small bottles of tonic with which they would place drops of liquid on patients' lips hoping that it would make a difference. And that's all they had. House calls were common, and the majority of the time spent between the physician and the patient was one of handholding, discussion, and listening. Oftentimes, "medicine" came down to simply offering comfort and above all a committed relationship.

The physician and the patient had a covenant relationship based on an understanding of who each other was, their roles, and what each could offer. There was no need to hide behind any lies because everyone knew each other. It is still remarkable to me that holding the hand of the patient was the common practice and the most prominent tool that the physician had. In today's world, physician and patient come together simply by chance and more often than not have no shared values. Insurance companies broker the relationship. When the physician and the patient come together it is done so by random selection. The chances of having shared values, shared virtues, shared interests, common backgrounds or communities are far from realistic.

We all know that within the first five to ten seconds of meeting someone new, we judge them as to whether we will like them or not, and we do so based on physical characteristics or physical values that we see and appreciate. After a short discussion we can pretty much tell whether we will have anything in common. Physicians need to move beyond that and to find a commonality between a patient and him in order to establish a covenant relationship. It's not hard to do. It's as easy as taking a moment to find a shared value. I tell my residents, find something that is of importance to you and your patient so that the relationship can move away from being a mere contract: a relationship based simply on a patient seeking a commodity of medicine and a physician offering that for a fee.

Instead, it is incumbent upon us to stop and ask the all-important, but very simple, questions: "Tell me a little bit about yourself. What do you do? What is a typical day like for you? How have things been going the last few weeks in your life, and are you having any stressful issues at this time?" Yes, you're setting yourself up to find out some very personal information, but it is information that can help you care better for your patient. It is important to distinguish the "who" from the "what." When you ask personal questions, you're finding out about the "who" of the patient, not the "what" of the health issue they're facing. For example, Let's take a patient who has an ulcer because he is stressed over money. In a contract relationship, you write a prescription for an antacid and think nothing more of it. However, the simple act of writing a prescription for an antacid is not necessarily the only thing that the patient is looking for. The physician's understanding of the cause of the abdominal pain and the fact that he or she has taken the time to listen and to explore more deeply the root cause of the abdominal pain is what the covenant relationship is all about. The simple act of "being present when present" is what makes the difference when it comes to a relationship.

I didn't learn this all overnight. In fact, I learned it from my patients. I deal with the issues of "care" every day, both comfort care and heroic care. Practicing pediatric critical care medicine embraces both. Children are admitted who are trying to die, or will die. Over the many years of practicing critical care medicine, I have learned that "caring" needs to be more than we give, and is frequently less than what patients receive. I deal with the issues of "care" over "cure" and life over death every day, and here is what I've found: it's about the "who," not about the "what."

There are times when we look at ourselves in the mirror and ask why we do what we do. Most of the time the answers are not what God wants to hear: "because we want to." When I go on a medical mission, it's not because I want to, but because I was asked to. He asked me to go. I didn't question why, I didn't ask how, and I never said no. I just did it. I overcame hurtles, obstacles, and spiritual warfare. I went and He led the way. It wasn't even a contest. He always won. Period.

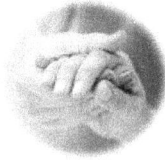

CHAPTER 11
DO YOU TREAT THE DISEASE OR THE PATIENT?

Before I discuss the need to treat the patient, not the disease, a general discussion of what constitutes a "disease" is in order. In the primordial state years ago, life was a continuum, for the most part uninterrupted. Health led to disease, which led to health again, or death, without intervention, nature directing the way. As medicine became sophisticated, interventional methods (both medicinal and technological) intervened with this continuum. Man now directed the way, and for the most part the outcome was in favor of the patient.

From a physiologic standpoint, the sick patient presents himself in a state of *entropy*, or a state of general disorder implying an illness or injury, and through a series of interventions, the patient returns to a healthy state or *homeostasis*. This process can also be blocked, as is seen with iatrogenic complications or physiologic setbacks.

The physiological state is related to the relative degree of health that the person has. Technology plays a more significant role as these physiologic states change. The body in its *normal* state functions by a series of complex interactions that are self-regulated, and its activities are crucial at maintaining this capacity. As the patient first gets ill, the body enters a *pre-disease* state. Organs have a tendency to malfunction, which is undetectable in the resting state but may appear when stress is applied. As the malfunction increases in magnitude, the body enters a *disease* state in which there is an uncoupling among the self-regulated feedback metabolic and physiologic cascades. The result is a physiologically chaotic state, one that grabs the attention of the scientific physician. The physician's purpose is to get the patient back to a state of homeostasis or wellness. In doing so, the disease becomes the focus of the physician's actions.

It seems that language directs and affects our actions. We want to be called something positive and unique. The "professional" has found its way into all niches of life, making all who want it "professionals." The *teacher* has become an educator. The *minister, rabbi,* and *priest* have become "clergy." The *patient* has become a customer or client. The *child* has become a "product." The *physician* has become a "healthcare provider." Here is an example of how disease has changed our focus and affected our language:

"This is a 10-year-old boy referred to us by his pediatric healthcare provider, who states that this client has new-onset diabetes mellitus. He is the product of a gravida 2 para 2 female with no family history of diabetes. The boy's educator at school informed the parents that he has been drifting off to sleep during class. The boy has also been acting out at home, and the parents sought help from their clergyman. He is here for education and a workup."

A more just and *person-oriented* presentation would be:

"John is a 10-year-old boy, who presents with new onset diabetes mellitus. He is the firstborn son of a gravida 2 para 2 mother, who states that she is unaware of any history of diabetes mellitus in her family. John's teacher has found him to be unusually tired at school, and he has been acting out at home. The parents sought help from their priest, who referred them to their physician, who in turn referred this patient, John, to our diabetic teaching center for diabetic teaching."

We begin to see the issue of desensitization. We are talking about "what," not "who." We refer to the boy as a "disease" and not by his name. We talk about a "case" that needs to be "worked up," not a patient that needs to be evaluated and examined. We talk about a "client," not a patient. The patient becomes the focus simply by recognizing him as a person entitled to such.

CHAPTER 12

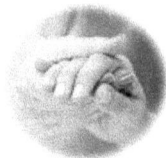

IS THE RELATIONSHIP BETWEEN THE PHYSICIAN AND THE PATIENT A CONTRACT OR A COVENANT?

One of the greatest tasks physicians have to face is to decide who they are, and what their relationship with their patient is going to be. As a result of something physicians do, are their patients better off?

Fueled by increased public knowledge and sophistication and necessitated by the overwhelming choices offered by technological advances, the movement for patient autonomy has come to the fore. Patients have become more aggressive in demanding a more active part in the decision-making process, and truth telling is expected but not always declared.

Four major developments over time have threatened to erode physicians' trustworthiness: 1) the use of financial incentives from healthcare organizations to limit care, 2) physicians investing in medical laboratories and other businesses to which they refer their patients posing a threat to physician trustworthiness by creating an incentive to order unnecessary tests, 3) the development of modern healthcare organizations through acquisitions and bundling resulting in patients having to switch physicians and endure shorter appointment visits and 4) doctors unaware of patients' advance directives or not having honest discussions with their patients during visits regarding wishes, goals and plans for the inevitable end of life.

Autonomy, the respect for self-determination, has made the doctor-patient relationship more horizontal. Doctor and patient make decisions on a more equalized basis. Medical care has evolved into a negotiated process rather than a physician-dictated plan of action. There is much good in the ascendancy of patient choice, but medical care has become more of a *contractual*, legalistic, rights-based agreement, which greatly diminished the trust that marked the old relationship between doctor and patient, the *covenant*. Through the centuries up until about thirty years ago, patients could be sure that their personal physician was truly their advocate and was always acting in their best interests—as healer when possible but always as a caring companion. Such assurance brought with it the confidence and trust that characterized the covenant relationship. Events of recent years have placed many external pressures on physicians, who find themselves increasingly accountable not only to their patients but also to insurance companies, Medicare, Medicaid, and to their hospital's quality assurance program and now by reputation based on quality reports. One can go to Angie's List to find a physician—no different than finding a plumber, contractor, or bricklayer. All of this with the very real specter of malpractice suits hanging over their heads. A contractual relationship implies success. If the patient does not recover from the illness, then someone is at fault, and malpractice becomes the norm. If we physicians seem distracted during our patient encounters, it is understandable because the patient's immediate problem is no longer our only worry. And the time pressures may concentrate our thoughts on the curing to the exclusion of the caring role. But this distraction also engenders patient doubt. "Is the doctor doing this test because he truly thinks I need it or because he has a financial interest in the testing facility?" Or, "Is the doctor not doing this test because she thinks I don't need it or because it will save the insurance company money?" All of this tends to diminish the warm, knowing, trusting relationship that once existed between doctor and patient, the covenant. The patient perceives this preoccupation as a lack of true interest and wonders, "Is this doctor really my friend and advocate?"

A true patient advocate must teach and inform the patient. Communication is the key—and communication skills were never more important. Modern healthcare has been described as a shared process—a partnership between the physician, who is an expert on medical matters, and the patient, who is an expert on what he or she wants.

For that shared process of decision making to take place,

patients must be carefully and accurately informed about all of the pertinent aspects of their illness and the preferred proposed treatment, and reasonable alternate treatments as well as the likely result of no treatment (for this always remains an option). Patients must understand that consent after provision of full information carries an obligation for them; they must then accept whatever risk is described and, if the outcome is less than perfect through no negligence of the physician, they must also be willing to accept that consequence. This is important to do when there is a contractual arrangement.

It is up to the physician to guide the patient so that expectations are reasonable and realistic. If quiet, thorough conversation achieves a full realization of the risks and benefits, the occasional less-than-optimal result may not seem so catastrophic.

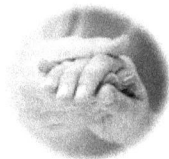

CHAPTER 13
IS YOUR PRIORITY CURING OR CARING?

The physician's task is to not only cure an illness, but to care for patients. One needs to act rightly at the right time for the right reasons in the right manner.

The "process" of care rather than the goal of care seems to be a primary intent of many physicians. We need to consider the intent versus the motive. The fact of the matter is that sometimes we don't care, we don't have time to care, we don't know how to care, and patients sometimes don't want caring. In the past, physicians had few effective means of treatment. The best they could do was to comfort the patient and wait for the disease to run its course. The patience and compassion served to comfort and heal the sick. Years ago, the patient was cared for by someone who served. As far as we know, the first physicians may have been priests. As knowledge was acquired, mystique became fact and physicians were born. But faith in the healer's skills persisted.

So when did caring get buried by curing? We need to

address the issues of care as they relate to cure first. Do patients receive the care they need? Do patients need the care they receive? In other words, as a result of something physicians do, are their patients better off? Today, patients are expected to recover. When they don't, then the assumption is that someone is at fault. Caring is skewed as a result. I challenge whether there is a difference between "caring about," "to take care of," and "to care for." Each demonstrates a different type of caring, and one could argue that one type of caring is significantly different than the other. How would you demonstrate each? Would it be related to time?

How one does is as important as *what* one does. When we have a covenant relationship, when we know who our patients are, our attitude is such that we begin to care, and with that caring comes compassion. We must become aware of our habits. What specific habits do you bring to the bedside? We need to have a clear idea about the chain that links our habits to patient-centered care. Which habits do you believe contribute to the quality care that outpatients receive? Which habits contribute to making people feel better? And which habits hinder patient care?

Caring encompasses the aspect of *humanism*. Although the definition of humanism is complex and wide, I will use the term to mean simply an unselfish compassion for another human being that becomes a way of life. Anything more raises expectations that are unreachable. It is unfortunate that humanism has lost part of its meaning. We recognize a deficiency in humanism by simply looking at changes in our culture: there is a growing plea for patient care advocates, patient bill of rights, and hospices for dying patients. The increased reports of humiliation experienced by clinicians when they themselves have been patients, and the emergence of autonomy rather than beneficence as the dominant principle in medical ethics supports a lack of a covenant relationship in today's medicine. In the physician's defense, humanism may be hard to come by. There may be unrealistic expectations that the patient imposes on the physician. Insurance companies who dictate patient care may direct the physician. Simply avoiding self-serving goals may be all that is needed to bring humanism to the bedside and with that comes compassion.

Reasons for avoiding compassion include conflict, resentment, and time, being uncomfortable with it, shunned, and not knowing how to offer it. Why is compassion more important now? There are several reasons:

- Lack of close-knit communities

- Lack of ready support of nearby relatives and friends

- Geographic distances between family members

Because of these reasons, physicians are expected to be more compassionate than they prefer to be. Compassion and caring may be common virtues held by all physicians. They cannot be taught but may at times need reinforcement and can be nurtured. Our society may be described by some as a pseudo-caring society, one that pretends to care but lacks sincerity. Witness the current trends both in business and family life: me first, you second. A caring environment is hard to come by. This may be directly related to a change in behavior that has occurred over a significant period of time that leads to a change in culture. If the majority holds to a certain behavior, the culture then becomes that behavior. In addition, physicians need feedback (nourishment) when caring; otherwise they get exhausted.

Differentiating between *curing* and *caring* can be argumentative indeed. In order to put them into perspective we need to make no pretense that both curing and caring are interchangeable, but they both can and should work in harmony. To do otherwise precludes a balanced approach to the patient. *Healing* and *healthcare* are also two very different processes, and are less inclined to work in harmony.

1. To **cure** implies to make better. It can be very objective and without emotion. A patient is sick and now he is cured—a relatively easy task to accomplish in most cases. It is the process of recovery or relief from a disease by instituting a treatment. Cure is a process of correction; objective in scope, objective in purpose. Curing promotes wholeness of body, a well-tuned machine.

2. **Healthcare** is intuitively objective and scientific. It encompasses a process and an institution.

3. **Healing** is more passionate, robust, and personal. It

encompasses the total well being of the person without boundaries.

4. **Caring** is the act of being present when present.

Caring is a personal matter. The physician and/or the patient may or may not be wanting or willingly able to care.
Caring can in fact be somewhat variable as it relates to an
attitude, feeling, or state of mind about a person and to a
particular skill that a person has. To care implies a much
more personal involvement by both the physician and the patient. Dr. Pellegrino eloquently described caring to me one
day when he said, "We need to have an understanding of
what sickness means to another person, together with the
readiness to help and to see the situation as the patient does.
Compassion demands that the physician be so disposed that
his every action and word will be rooted in respect for the
person he is serving." He wrote about this many times. He
started me thinking about the notion of being present when
present with my patients.

I see *caring* as a process of promoting wholeness of being which embraces three aspects of humanism that I believe
serve as common denominators for all physicians: to prevent
and control pain, to ensure the patient's comfort, and to maintain his dignity.

Cure	Caring	Healthcare	Healing
Fix	Empathy	Insurance	Whole
Healthy	Touch	Hospital	Holistic
Better	Listen	System/ administration	Involvement
Attention	Being present when present	Process/ procedures	Personal

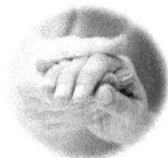

CHAPTER 14
CASEY AND TECHNOLOGY

The next step in my journey towards understanding what a covenant is, happened almost as an afterthought. I remember Casey as a tender child. I can't quite tell whether it was force of personality or the fact that he was irresistibly affectionate that attracted him to me. Overall, he was not unlike all the other children we see in the pediatric critical care unit. Not to imply that this little person was generic in any sense, but he was at least no different in acuity and the disease process than what we are used to.

Casey was almost four years old and had Hurler's syndrome, a rare genetic disorder that causes the liver and spleen to enlarge, respiratory problems, as well as physical and mental retardation. The internal difficulties generally prove fatal at a very early age. Casey and his entire life consisted of hospitalizations for treatment of worsening respiratory distress. His mental handicap left him unable to properly communicate his wants and needs, but those who knew him understood. He was clearly tired but remained courageous. Daily patient rounds consisted of the reiteration of a problem list that remained unchanged for days, and "status quo" was the terminology commonly used as the days progressed. All of us in the critical care unit were quick to discuss the pathophysiology of this patient's disease, but evaded the most important topic because we lacked the courage to seek full knowledge of Casey's life.

On many occasions I observed otherwise rational, intelligent individuals extolling the virtues of bringing in more consultants and increasing the level of technological support, for no other reason than to do something to this child. The dreadful irony of the whole thing was that I began to establish a relationship with the family and the child while simultaneously encouraging the proliferation of layers of science and technology that would serve no purpose other than to isolate the patient and family further from each other and me.

Something clearly was wrong.

I was either afraid of the patient and his family or the disease itself. Over the course of several weeks, Casey deteriorated, and the family struggled with hopes and disappointments that rocked them from side to side until they could no longer stand strong. Details aside, it was agreed to let Casey die. He was made comfortable with morphine and was in his mother's arms when he died. That day signaled a time for reflection—something I had not done much of up to that point.

I had entered this situation with a conviction that displayed uncertainty and a degree of trepidation, and as I pondered that, it became clear to me for the first time there is a need for a balance between what some call "High Tech" and "High Touch."

As I reflected on Casey's treatment, I realized that we have a pattern in modern medicine. As the patient gets sicker the balance tips in favor of "high tech," and "high touch" falls away. Perhaps we would all agree that there should be a balance between the two, but it is too easy to push "high tech" and avoid "high touch." We're fighting for our patients' lives. Time seems to be a major factor and there isn't enough of it to go around. Medicine is not such a cut-and-dried affair that it is not uninhabited by fads and fashions. It is fashionable these days to comment or perhaps to lament about the way physicians look at their own approach to "high tech" and "high touch." I am pleased to say that a general awareness has emerged that physicians must be more caring. But I want that to be more than just a fad.

Looking back, I think that we have always been, but our focus has been blurred. There is so much to know of the human condition and we understand so little. However, the human spirit accepts challenge, and there appear to be alternatives for those daring enough to pursue them.

With Casey, I was forced to ask two of the questions I've posed: do we treat diseases or do we treat patients, and is the technology we use a necessity for the patient or as a convenience for us? Uncertainty shapes the decisions made by physicians daily. Yes, there are often decisions made based on bona fide, documented test results or a good physical examination. But for the most part, the approach to the disease process is one of defense. Modern medicine may be pointed in the wrong direction by focusing on treating the disease rather than addressing the suffering it sometimes causes the patient. Physicians are no more or no less honest than other persons, but the structure of the subject imposes a demand for adherence to a set of rigid rules that keeps the structure intact. Physicians must see symptoms in context of the patient's whole life and person.

My relationship with Casey and his parents evolved from a realization that we can't take time for granted, and we must underscore the importance of "high touch." I had a stark realization that day Casey died. Letting children like Casey die without suffering or watching the sick child heal and live bring the same rewards only if we put "high touch" and "high tech" in balance. We need to think honestly when using "high tech." Is its purpose a necessity or a convenience?

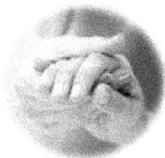

CHAPTER 15
IS THE TECHNOLOGY WE USE A NECESSITY OR A CONVENIENCE?

The momentum in technology growth yielded an environment driven by "modern" doctors who chose to use technology to drive patient care. The question asked therefore is, is the technology used today a necessity or simply a convenience? In other words, is the technology invaluable in giving accurate answers to questions that would be otherwise unobtainable by other means, and therefore contribute directly to patient care, or is it used solely as a convenience for the clinician so that they can attend to other things? This has become evident by a diagnostic revolution that took place over a period of 100 years. Technology was recognized as a potential deterrent to patient care back in the late 1800s when S. Meir Mitchell said in a presidential address to the Congress of American Physicians and Surgeons: "You know, alas! That we now use as many instruments as a mechanic does." (*Boston Medical and Surgical Journal* September 24, 1891 Volume 125 No 13 page 311)

It should not be misconstrued that I am taking an anti-technology posture. Not at all. I believe that the advances in medicine have come about as a direct result of this very technology. It is, however, this technological *knowledge* that must become technological *wisdom* in order for it to be used appropriately.

Medicine is addicted to technology. We are infatuated with its remarkable engineering, its prowess, and its mystique. Medicine has become a science of machines, with less and less of the human touch that was once the foundation for healing. This "high touch" has become overshadowed by "high tech." Technology has progressed to the point where it at times supersedes caring, implying a type of pseudo-caring that can leave the patient isolated and empty. Often as the patient gets sicker, the use of technology goes up and the human interaction between clinician and patient goes down. This depersonalization is inconsistent with the purpose of medicine and forces the escalation of unnecessary high-tech interventions that cause human suffering. The foundational premise of *primum non nocere* encompasses the basic principles of avoidance of harm. Technology has caused iatrogenic events that go against the benefit of the patient. This iatroepidemic is morally unacceptable.

On the other hand, technology has opened windows into the disease process that has allowed many human lives to be saved. Technology can be a powerful adjunct to the clinician's expertise, and the standard of care in modern medicine expects its use. The proper use of technology in a critical care environment should be based on a foundation of humanism. Technology has at times taken away from the humanistic approach to the patient so that clinicians have become more comfortable treating the disease rather than the patient and more comfortable with curing than with caring. Consider this: 1) whether there is, or can be, a balance between the use of technology and compassion at the bedside, and 2) how can technology be made to be more humane and 3) what is of primary interest to the patient. Is it the assurance of patient comfort and patient dignity, i.e., humanism?

Technology in its narrowest sense is a tool or material artifact that assists in a task. By its design and its particular use, technology can be less than neutral in its application. A hammer can be used to build a house or bash in a head. By design, the hammer is supposed to be used as an instrument to pound nails, not heads. Once the artifact is used contrary to its design, it becomes an instrument of questionable purpose. Technology cannot be neutral. It constitutes a way of life and human behavior.

Technology changes behavior and culture by virtue of having the ability to change the environment. This change comes as a result of trying to resolve a particular problem, but often it replaces that problem with another. Technology has overpowered patients and healthcare providers alike. Rarely does the patient in the critical care unit give informed consent for the use of technology. The question is not whether technology is good or bad, but whether it is used appropriately and with humane intentions.

Technology threatens to deprive the patient of freedom by being restrictive and invasive. It can also expand freedom by giving access and mobility (wheelchair). Finding a balance between the two seems to be difficult since technology has little tolerance for balance. Technology is a crutch for the poor clinician and an adjunct for the good one.

The behavior of a physician is related to the conditions under which he lives and practices. Technology has desensitized the physician from covenant relationships and we see that in all aspects of our society: texting, rather than talking face to face or picking up a phone; Facebook posts to tell everyone we are going shopping; selfies that showcase the "me"; and e-mails rather than writing letters.

The human touch seems to fall by the wayside when the patient gets sicker. The more ill the patient becomes, the more technology is used. There is a gap between high tech and high touch. The patient is lost in an ocean of machines, medicines, and consultants. The clinician becomes a conductor of a technological orchestra, much of which is out of tune with the patient. Technology has developed its own momentum in medicine without respect for the patient's dignity, comfort, and worth. Clinical diagnosis has been replaced by technological diagnosis. Technology has perhaps been too successful. Through research and development based on presumptive needs of the patient, new technology is developed. This high tech in turn causes an increase in the public's expectation, which leads to an increase in the physician's need to use high tech, which then leads to further high-tech development. It has assumed a dominate position in medicine and may lead to its own destruction by becoming so unyielding that it destroys personal choice. The thrust of technology has reduced patients to organized systems and can become more important than the patient it was designed to serve. Technology should come as a result of a genuine understanding of the disease process, the limitations of the clinician, and the patient's best interest.

The current question of the role and value of technology is nothing new. There is no question that technology is an essential component of modern medicine. Technology has been invaluable in giving clinicians a window into areas of the human body inaccessible by the routine physical examination, and it has given the clinician an early look at the disease process. But the rate of technological change has developed its own momentum with innovations that are increasing at an accelerated rate sometimes without respect for patient comfort, needs, wants, or dignity. By using technology as a substitute for our personal intervention with patients, we force distance between the patients and ourselves. We are who we are as a result of technological changes. We have come to depend on them and accept them as a way of life. Technology has taken out the human, personal mechanics of life that once drove our cultures: picking crops by hand, now by machine, doing math by reason, pencil, and paper, now by computer, and palpating pulses with fingers, now by Doppler and infrared technology and using an echocardiogram to evaluate a heart rather than using our stethoscopes. I sense some pushback here and I will admit that technology has and will give us information that we are unable to obtain without it, that it has given us the opportunity to "look inside" the body at the macro and micro level, and has given us the opportunity to predict the likelihood of having or getting a disease (genetic testing, translational research, genome sequencing and more). But have we asked the hard questions that need to be answered before we implement the technology? Is the patient and the physician prepared to address the consequences of a positive breast cancer marker in a 15-year-old female? When do we tell her and when should she be told she will get breast cancer, and that a bilateral mastectomy is the best course of action within the next few years before the cancer appears? Technology has sparked a significant cause of social change. There should be no technological imperative, or a "one best way." There needs to be human choices. Some of these choices may be ethical in nature, and we ask who will make them and for whom will they be made? Technology has forced us to look at "what," and not the "who." Using high technology forces the issue of man as machine. Patients become cases that are worked up. Technology allows the physician to distance himself from the patient. If the physician and the patient's eyes can't meet, there is a problem. In using technology, physicians mistakenly believe they can reduce uncertainty by changing the patient's problem to one in which there is a technological answer.

Technology assessment at the bedside is also lacking. Some clinicians erroneously believe that technology always gives the right answer. In fact, physicians use technology convinced of its success, fueled by the promise of performance rather than performance itself. Technology threatens a quality of life that requires a freedom of choice and a right to comfort and dignity. The information that technology yields may not necessarily transfer to better patient care. In fact, we have seen that some technology is incapable of contributing anything of meaning to better the patient. Technological abuse occurs not infrequently in critical care. Tests may be performed when none are warranted. Some causes of technological abuse involve physicians' motivation, such as a desire for profit, desire for enhanced prestige in an academic setting, desire to experience a fascination or pleasure associated with a new procedure, and the simple desire for self-protection when possible against legal action. Harsh words you say. I agree, but words truthful all the same and certainly not for all physicians.

There are two assumptions that need clarification: first, that technology implies better patient outcomes, and second, the physician and the patient need technology. Technology has become a way of life. Technology may in fact compromise patient outcome by prolonging illness and death. Technology should simply allow the clinician and the patient to work more closely together in the healing process. When used appropriately, technology yields exciting information that contributes directly to an immediate action by the clinician and improvement of patient outcome. One example is the test for cholesterol. A simple test allows the clinician to use the information to prescribe a therapy that may lower the cholesterol, thus improving patient outcome. It implies that the test can reasonably determine a course of therapy that for the most part will benefit the patient. High tech becomes unnecessary if it has no benefit to or for the patient.

Technology can prolong the inevitable—a death that may be hard to come by. It can be this very use of technology that undermines the essence of medicine by obstructing a process that cannot be changed. Technology, on the other hand, can push away death, ensuring normal survival. Deciding when to use technology is founded in the determination by the patient, family, and the physician as to the best guess for outcome. Technology will always be a means for creating new physical and human conditions by interfering in a natural process. Even in everyday life, we see technology used in contrast to nature: air-conditioning for summer heat and artificial heat for winter cold. At the same time, there is argument for the very use of technology in life. The mere existence of technology dictates that it be used. It will also always have the potential to destroy the essence of humanism.

I take the hard road if only to bring light to the danger

of using technology as a crutch rather than as an adjunct to our skills as physicians. I believe in technology even though it may not seem that way. I just ask that we make sure that technology does not trump the very essence of the physician-patient relationship.

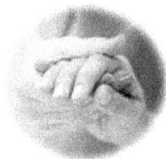

CHAPTER 16
HIGH-TECH COMPANIES: RESPONSIBILITIES

In the world of medical technology, professional engineers and managers claim to make a contribution to medicine by developing technology that helps clinicians care for the patient. Clinicians are the customers of the company. I argue that the high-tech company has the wrong "customer" and that the company as a whole contributes little to patient care. In developing technology, they ask the clinicians what their needs are. The company should be asking patients what their needs are. An analogy would be as follows: An author of a grade-school mathematics book writes the text with the student in mind: the child's age, level of understanding, language skills, and needs. The author does not write the text for the teacher. The teacher is simply a user of the text. The author writes for the student. In medical technology today, the instrument is developed for the clinician, not the patient. Technology should be patient driven. Today, the great majority of technology is in search of a patient. Rather than developing technology to fit the patient's needs, the patient is being required to fit technology's mold.

Physicians seem to serve technology with more reverence than toward their patients. Physicians tend to become mediators between patient and technology. Physicians become more reluctant to use their clinical skills and rely on their use of technology for cure. Humanizing technology should start by recognizing the patient as the person for whom technology is used. If we agree that technology can directly affect a patient's comfort, dignity, and autonomy, we perhaps should consider the patient as the center of technology. High-tech companies continue to develop technology that may or may not meet the needs of the patient. In the evolution of critical care, the emphasis has been on technology and practices of cure rather than on the patient-physician relationship. That is cure over care. Technology then follows by driving cure at the expense of care. There should be a balance where the patient has a comfort level of knowing that technology is helping with more accurate monitoring and diagnosis and the patient has a comfort level that he trusts and relies on the physician for care.

In the past, physicians had few effective means of treatment. The best they could do was to comfort the patient and wait for the disease to run its course. The patience, compassion, and faith in this role served to comfort and heal the sick. Years ago, the patient was cared for by someone who served. I suggest that high-tech companies and clinicians alike consider the following: patient-centered care as a stepping-stone to a more sound foundation: human-centered care. By looking at patients as humans, we will be reminded of our intentions: humane caring.

Technology impacts on human values (respect for the worth of another human being). It has taken the burden of caring off our backs and our minds. We have no need to think and in some cases have made decision making unnecessary. Perhaps this should bother us.

In each complex critically ill patient, several pathogenic processes may be present, each having its own likelihood of resulting in death and its own probability of reversal with critical care support. Faced with a choice between using technology and using compassion to treat these pathogenic processes, we strive to find a balance between the two. Technology is supposed to minister to human needs. Instead, addictive as it is, it tends to weigh heavy in patient care. The patient becomes the object of technology.

Clinicians and patients may not necessarily need technology to live or die, but simply to allow the clinician and the patient to work more closely together in the healing process. Curing is certainly our goal, but caring should be our passion.

For technology companies, there is an increasing struggle to balance the patient's best interest and the bottom line. High-tech companies need to accept the responsibility for the appropriate development of technology. They also should be looking at their "caring principles": are they doing what they should be doing, or are they bounding their efforts by what they can do? Are we focusing on the development of optimal solutions for the use of technology or just alternative solutions that may or may not lead to the optimal solution? Physicians need to define the minimum information needed to achieve an optimal clinical outcome. Who is to construct the technological environment and to what end? Who will use a technology and to what end? Physicians practice in accordance with a built-in set of caring values which direct their character and practice style. On the other hand, technology has had a direct impact on our values by its capacity for creating new opportunities and by making possible what was not possible before. It offers new options to choose from. However, we must be careful not to allow principles to be replaced by utility.

It is our responsibility to ensure the appropriate use of technology by education and understanding that technology reflects human power and also weakness. In trying to solve the technological problems facing us, we should turn to the things we do best. We should play from strength, and our strengths are our characters and principles as physicians. Humanism leads the way. Simply, as a result of something we do, are patients better off?

We need a rethinking of the kind of physician we really want to be. We need to ask ourselves who we are from the patient's point of view. We need to ask who we are in relationship to our patients. We need to identify technology "abuse." We must find a balance between high tech and high touch.

We must ensure that patients drive technology and not high technology or even clinicians.

How is the clinician to decide if the use of technology is a convenience or a necessity? Asking whether the technology to be used is a necessity or a convenience will lead to a better relationship between clinician and patient. Is there a surplus of technology? The critical care unit should not be expected to be a high-tech setting, but rather should be expected to be a haven in which humane care is delivered. I suggest that if high tech substitutes for caring by becoming the dominant principle in patient care, then it becomes pseudo-caring.

Technology should only be used to support life if appropriate, as an adjunct to care, and as a replacement for an injured organ system (necessity). Technology should not be used if it becomes biased towards the clinician, benefits the clinician over the patient, and limits the patient's interaction with the caregiver (convenience). Technology should come as a result of a genuine understanding of the disease process, the limitations of the clinican, and the patient's best interest.

I pose more questions than offer answers. However, by addressing these questions we will force the issue of humanizing technology.

- Just because we are capable of an action such as technology, should we do it?

- Who should control emerging technology: high-tech companies, clinicians, patients, or society?

- What types of studies are necessary to validate a particular technology's usefulness?

- What type of informed consent is necessary for the use of technology?

- Do clinicians have an obligation to inform the patients about uncertainty of the benefits of a particular technology?

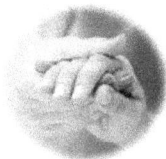

CHAPTER 17
COVENANTS AND BOB

Dore Schary an American producer once said that "the portrait of a man is a fusion of what he thinks he is, what others think he is, what he really is, and what he tries to be". I believe we all fit that description very nicely. But interestingly enough, as physicians, our portraits have been painted in neon, a glaring flashing light, as compared to the subtle pastel colors of most other people, and of course there is a reason for that. It seems that we are expected to always be something we perhaps can't or don't know how to be. We are expected to be above all kind, loving, gentle, compassionate, caring, and sensitive. I would challenge that I expect the same from my fellow human beings—physician or not. Since that is not always so, and since we sometimes feel cheated by always giving and receiving nothing in return, we have a tendency to become strangers at the bedside. We are strangers to our patients and we are strangers to their families. Being a stranger brings with it a lack of trust and mutual respect. It is so much easier that way. And no health-care provider bound by culture, religion, or race is immune.

The issue came to light one day. Bob had been struggling all day trying to breathe and finally made his way to the critical care unit, where ventilation seemed inevitable and not very comforting. He had cystic fibrosis, and for seventeen years of his life he had learned to live with the labored breathing, the lack of oxygen, and the dependency on others to help him stay alive. He had arrived at the end of a long road—no exit, no rest stop, and no opportunity to make a U-turn. As I explained to Bob what I was about to do, I was struck by his labored voice asking me to hurry. As the nurses got ready and the ventilator rolled into the room, Bob asked for some private time with his father. Bob and his dad whispered in each other's ear, hugged, kissed, and passed pictures back and forth, hurriedly reliving precious moments they had shared. A few short minutes later I put Bob on a ventilator, knowing that doing so would possibly never see him come off.

Just a few days before I put Bob on the ventilator, Bob and his girlfriend were supposed to go to the prom, but because Bob was in the hospital, some creative arrangements were necessary. Bob's hospital room became their banquet hall, his girlfriend came dressed in splendor fitting the occasion, they ate, and Bob self-consciously quickly took off his oxygen to pose for pictures. I left the room feeling intrusive, a stranger, but was called back. "Doctor, you're needed in Bob's room." Not David, not Doctor Beyda, but just "doctor." I really don't remember the first time I was called "doctor" and not that it matters, but you would think that it would have warranted a special place in my memory bank considering I worked long and hard to earn the title. Being called "doctor" several times a day for years had made me immune to the portrait it implied. It served as a reminder of the "what" (a doctor), not the "who" (a silent servant).

I entered the room not knowing what to expect. I was asked of nothing, however, except for my presence. As I stood there, I began to understand their needs and more importantly, Bob's need. I had role models before me, unrecognized until now, and I quickly learned. Bob's family, nurses, and other staff were there with him until the very end. I should be there too. In the current medical model, it is too easy for us to leave. We're strangers at the bedside. I posed a question of myself at that very moment, and found an answer in the people around me.

Four days after I put Bob on the ventilator, I took him off and allowed him to die with his parents, sister, and friends in attendance. The same pictures shared earlier and which were particularly difficult to look at for me were passed around to Bob's friends, who came to visit as they said good-bye.

∽∞∽

There is a difference between curing and caring. There is a definite difference between healing and healthcare. Yes, people who are sick like to be cured. Curing implies a scientific approach to the patient with a successful recovery as its end. Caring, on the other hand, has nothing to do with science, success, recovery, or intervention. Healthcare implies a means to cure. Healing implies acceptance, dignity, and comfort. I have found myself sometimes emphasizing cure at the expense of caring. Although some would argue that we do in fact care, I argue that we have produced extended resources to cure diseases and few to take care of patients.

Our neon portrait shows us as curing healthcare providers who are strangers to our patients. We perhaps would rather be caring healers, companions to our patients whether in suffering or wellness. We have been empowered to comfort by virtue of our vocation. I chose not to use the word *work*. Healing is not a career. It is a covenant we choose to believe in and to accept, and with that, there is no room for strangers at the bedside.

Physicians, most believe, are supposed to cure people. Curing is relatively easy. Caring is burdensome. Healthcare is science. Healing is an art. We need to hear our patients and most importantly we need to listen. At the very least, we need to look seriously at what we do and who we are. We need to do what we should do and not what we can do. With Bob I had certainly failed as a curing healthcare provider. But was I able to do more, give more? It reminded me, for all that it matters, that even though I had been practicing medicine for years and was an expert technician, I was still not that caring, healing doctor who would be able to give a little more to my patients. To care about and to care for my patients. "Taking care of" patients is what we do. It takes a commitment, sometimes bold and courageous, to go beyond that, to look past the "what," the disease, and "care about" and "care for" the patient. The covenant part of the physician-patient relationship.

When Bob died, I had a sense of great loss, not because I had known him well and therefore would miss him, but because I realized that he had so much to offer, most of which was yet unborn. As I watched him pass away, I remembered the words that Oliver Wendell Holmes wrote: "for those who never sing, but die with all their music in them."

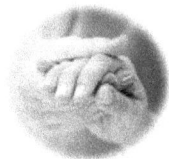

CHAPTER 18
MY UNCLE

What about our everyday tasks? The "doing" part of our job. I am often called upon to "prepare" my patients' families for the inevitable arrival of death. When my uncle died, I was given a stark reminder that there are other, bigger issues that must be faced as well.

The last time I saw my uncle alive, he was in a hospice, four days before he died. A brain tumor found a few short months before had rapidly debilitated him despite aggressive surgery and radiation. The diagnosis had been made quickly and without fanfare shortly after a routine visit to an ophthalmologist revealed papilledema—swelling in the back of the eye.

I was at his side in pre-op holding the day he went to have his baseball-size brain tumor removed. I listened to his speech slur as the Valium took effect and held his hand as he joked about waking up from surgery with a zipper in his head. He never once asked about the seriousness of what he had and he never showed anger or fear. It seemed like he took it for granted that this was part of life. I felt his courage as he squeezed my hand as he fought back the fear and anger.

Courage is sometimes misleading. There is the courage it takes to face a dangerous situation. There's courage in working in a place where people die all the time. But there is a different kind of courage: the courage to make oneself responsible for an outcome. My uncle had lived a wonderful life, unpretentious and filled with the happiness and love that he found in everyone and everything.

My uncle had always been special to me, and he was the favorite of all the nieces and nephews. Being a joker, he had a disposition that drew laughter and happiness all around him. He loved life for no other reason than to love it. He had a genius for being himself.

My aunt, not one of medical expertise, but one of persistent inquiry, strove to find the best care available, to do the very best to make him comfortable, and to challenge the very essence of dying. She was also very adept, I discovered, in making sure that her feelings never interfered with the care of my uncle. Because of the circumstances, telephone marathons between my aunt and me became the norm. She and I were never close, but we formed a bond that involved my uncle. We spoke of life and death, of pain and fear, of the right to die and the right to let go. We spoke of what my uncle would want if he were bedridden and dying. We never really came out and asked my uncle. It seemed as if he had dissolved himself of all his thoughts and left his determination to someone else.

After months of sharing feelings and thoughts, both objective and subjective, I felt that I had done a pretty good job of preparing my aunt for the time when my uncle would die. I deal with this task on a regular basis, and after many years of talking to parents about their dying children and preparing them for the moment of death, I likened myself to some sort of expert counselor. An advisor. Someone who brought solace to the grieving family. I had spent months guiding her, preparing her. I left no detail out. I described worst-case scenarios, the moment of death, and what she would possibly feel.

As we sat and talked in the few days that remained of my uncle's life, I asked a question that I asked frequently of family members, expecting an obvious answer: "He's going to die soon. Are you ready?"

Without hesitation she said, "When you love somebody, you're never ready."

This felt like a glass of cold water being thrown in my face to wake me up. For that's what it was. A wake-up call. If this is how she felt, I certainly have not come close with the families of my patients. She struck the heart of common sense. Of reality.

When my aunt gave me her simple answer, it forced me to ask myself what I had hoped to achieve when talking to parents, when asking them what I thought was the "final" question.

The answer I couldn't ignore. It is not simply that I do too much, but that I do so for the wrong reasons. Instead of just quiet support and acceptance, I force the issue of "being ready" for death. Because if parents are "ready," then physicians are absolved.

As physicians, our main task has always been to "diagnose." It's almost textbook: recognition of a specific illness based on what has been learned about the past history and any pathologic changes will lead the physician to an accurate diagnosis. From there, the doctor can forecast the likely outcome. And all this has to be explained to the patient. What the ill patient and the family wants most to know is the name of the illness, what possibly could have caused it, and finally, most important of all, what will eventually happen in a kind and gentle manner.

The rapidity with which illness, injury, and death present themselves is unquestionably frightening. Dwelling on what I should do to prepare parents, what I used to do, made me forget that I often felt like I needed to do more, but let it go as something nebulous and unimportant. I had so much to learn.

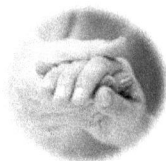

CHAPTER 19
DOCTOR NADAS

I'll never forget meeting Dr. Alexander Nadas. We sat outside, he reading the Sunday *New York Times*, I speaking every so often, but mostly sitting, waiting for an opportunity to say something. He commanded a presence of respect and dignity, not only because of his reputation, but also because of his unquestionable commitment to medicine. Dr. Nadas, known by all as a leader in the field of pediatric cardiology, was essentially holding court and it was my turn to be seen. I was there because some of what we do in medicine is based on tradition, and that tradition is based on the personal experience and the charisma of the leaders in the field. I wanted to talk to him about the issues of "care" versus "cure." I wanted him to know that this is a strange period in medicine. I wanted him to know that we are so twisted up in the business of medicine that we have lost our center.

What made it all so interesting was the difference in how we each perceived caring. We shared stories and perceptions about the way medicine was practiced years ago and how it is practiced today. He would on occasion look up from his paper, but most of the time he would talk while reading. I quickly learned when it was time for me to speak. When he turned a page, I went for it. I felt like a first-year medical student and then it hit me. His was a decidedly old-fashioned, paternalistic style. It was evident even in his thoughts and mannerisms.

He declared, more often than not, that the patient needs to be told what is to be done. He believed that the physician held the responsibility and the burden of making the patient better, and that the physician was the only one who could. I wanted to argue that this viewpoint was what got us into trouble in the first place, but then he said something that made me stop. He believed that nurses were better at caring than physicians. This is the thing that got me thinking.

He never said that physicians didn't care. He simply said that nurses did it better. I welcomed the debate and gave him a stack of my essays to read, hoping they would find their way to somewhere in between the editorial page and the book review section. He called me from Boston very late one night to ask a simple question: "Why do you have to write about such things? Doctors can't be doctors if they can't care." I mumbled something about a change in priorities and technological advances and that's when he hung up.

What moves me now as I think about what he said was that I was slow to realize the glaring truth of his words. We're supposed to care and care deeply. But how?

The next day, I went to the hospital. I had two patients, Keith and Brandon, both different but both very much the same. Both were on life support, high tech, medicine needed to support blood pressure and heart rate, and without all of that they would die. To each and for each, I took care of, cared for, and cared about. If it hadn't been for Keith and Brandon, I would never have begun to understand the question. While Brandon was in the unit, I knew him only as my patient, though he was always an unconventional one. Even the way he died was unconventional. He died by committee—multiple consultants' input from extended family members and clergy, all having a vote in his death. I couldn't help but notice it was simply a negotiated death brought about by a dying process that was not allowed to happen.

It disturbed me because it was clearly a dehumanizing process, a close kin to the other dehumanizing aspects of medicine today, when patients are referred to as clients, and physicians and nurses are called healthcare providers. I apologize for always referring to the ones who die, but they seem to be the ones who teach me the most, perhaps because I spend the time looking for answers to questions posed as they pass. But at the same time, the more lives I look into, the more I realize the incompleteness of the picture of medicine. We attempt to prevent compassion and caring for the sick person from getting lost in the enthusiasm for scientific medicine by trying to be more altruistic. I have come to realize that it is not about technology; it's about our culture. We try to do what is best, but find ourselves burdened by behavioral norms that have a skewed notion of what "best" is.

"Cure as well as care" is taken for granted as a fact of life. What then do we mean when we say I "care about you"? Is it different from I "care for you"? What about "taking care of you"? Either way, caring should occur simply, spontaneously, and without effort. Decisions made by physicians for and about their patients are increasingly being driven by outcomes data and the need to cure.

I begin to pose one of the questions many of you are now familiar with: I could save (cure), I would save (cure), but should I (care)? I sometimes deride myself because I am too busy to concern myself with anything but the present. I do notice however, families and friends at the bedside sharing an unconditional caring and compassion, far from the transparent forms I occasionally see. I see some of these families again from time to time. It seems that we have invested a little bit of ourselves in each other's lives. We discover that it has appreciated over the years—more than either of us could have expected. They make me realize how little I really know about myself and how little I understand the process of caring for my patients.

But reality hits home fairly hard. Keith's mother asked me a simple question. "How can Keith die, even if he wanted to?" It was simply a question of whether we would let him die or not. So true. The technology would not let him unless I turned it all off. The simple answer is that the economics of medicine and the trends towards cure will answer that scientific question. Finding the caring answer, however, is hard to do. We should and must be ready to examine ourselves critically, and when necessary, ask the hard questions that may not always produce happy answers.

This ethos of caring is something we strive to embrace, but find hard at times to understand. Perhaps Dr. Nadas could help. I waited until the middle of the week to call him hoping he'd be finished with the paper by then. He wasn't. I was on my own.

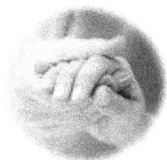

CHAPTER 20
MY FRIEND

His eyes, which I had remembered as penetrating, now appeared deeper set and very sad. I could not look into them for very long without feeling the pain and hurt that he was going through. A tragic event had disrupted his life, and I had come for no other reason than to be one of many who would try to explain why and to offer comfort if possible. It seems that through pain and tragedy, the best comes out in people and sometimes it stays, but for the most part it leaves only to return at another time. It was this event that forced the issue of deliberation. Am I who I should be or who I want to be? The answer lies in my own happiness. Unhappiness has been best described as the difference between our talents and expectations, and for the most part, I have a large gap between the two. This in no way implies a failure of character on my part, but rather a realistic appreciation of what I am. Like it or not, I am mediocre at best, or as Somerset Maugham once said, "the mediocre are always at their best." In medicine, mediocrity is not accepted. In life, it is the norm. The more lives I look into, the more I realize the truth of this matter.

It took many different experiences with patients for me to fully comprehend the importance of a covenant relationship with my patients. When this good friend and colleague lost a loved one in a very tragic accident. It made me question again my purpose as a doctor and what role a covenant plays in the doctor/patient relationship.

In medicine, we expect ourselves to excel and in fact it is demanded of us. At the same time, we argue that we are human, and as such, are prone to mistakes and lapses in excellence. If we were truly talented, as some of the great medical progenitors of long past were, then expectations would be met consistently and without effort. Comforting a patient, a colleague, or a family member is a natural talent we all possess. In this case, it was natural for me to be there with him. He and I talked, saying nothing but sharing much. What struck me was that it was important that there was a need to be there with and for each other. It was easy with us: two physicians, finding it easy to care and comfort each other. Why was it so hard for those same two physicians to care and comfort their patients? I found the answer in his eyes. We try too hard.

His eyes told me that what I was about to give was wanting, but more importantly, would I continue to give anyway? Our patients ask the same. I realized that we too often forget to answer. My time with my friend helped me to understand that to be able to comfort and care always, consistently, and unselfishly is a talent we would like to have, but as I reflected on it later, I also understood, with loathing in my heart, that we have a tendency to prevent compassion and caring for each other and our patients by being lost in the enthusiasm of our own needs and for scientific medicine. Sometimes it just does not work.

The sad fact is, our attitudes are such that we have changed from a giving society to one that takes. The sense of personal values and relationships with people has fallen by the wayside. It is business as usual. In medicine it is no different. Nurses don't have patients anymore; they have assignments. Patients aren't patients anymore; they are clients. With this new attitude, it is difficult to care.

As men and women of science, we hold ourselves above the questioning attitude of some who say we are superficial and portray a character that lacks meaning and sincerity. I now argue that point. It is not that we are insincere. What my friend ultimately helped me to understand, as my aunt did with my uncle's death, is that our sincerity in caring is at times transparent and ritualistic. Unquestionably, these are hard words written. However, we should and must be ready to examine ourselves critically, and when necessary, ask the hard questions that may not always give us the answers we want.

If it had not been for my taking the time to care for my

friend, I would never have asked those questions myself. But I ask them now, demanding answers of myself all the time, and I'm still seeking those answers.

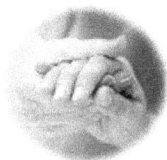

CHAPTER 21
KARI

Sometime long ago, I had my wrists well and truly slapped by a ten-year-old girl with trisomy 18—a lethal congenital abnormality caused by an extra eighteenth chromosome. Most children die in infancy from the complications.

Her name was Kari. She was admitted seriously ill with chicken pox and in a coma with little hope of recovery. The fact that she had trisomy 18 immediately "labeled" her as someone not in need of aggressive therapy and, therefore, received care that allowed her comfort but was far less than the mega-aggressive approach we would have given to a "normal" child. At the time, it seemed like a good plan.

Meeting Kari's mother for the first time, I prepared myself for the gibe I was about to receive. I expected to meet a mother with a fixed expression on her face that said, "Don't even try to imagine what I've seen or been through in the last ten years." Truth be told, she was delightful, and I was embarrassed. She was sincerely cordial and attentive. She placed no burden on me to accept the fact that Kari was special because she had outlived the medical profession's prophecy of an early death. What she did ask me for was to ensure Kari's comfort and dignity. Her request made me snap to attention. This amazing woman expressed a foresight that gave me the missing piece in my theory of covenant relationships.

When Kari was born, her parents were told that she would not live more than a few days. The family grieved and waited. Kari's mother recounts the rest.

"We waited, day after day, for Kari to die. She surprised us after the first week when she became easier to handle and feed. We gradually began to accept that Kari was in fact going to live, and we should make the best of it." Stroking Kari's forehead, she paused for a moment. "We...I, have lived with Kari for the past ten years with the same philosophy...that every day Kari lives, is a bonus...a gift...for which we are very thankful."

Kari's family incorporated her into their daily lives. With special effort, they were able to achieve a comfortable norm. Rather than trying to find ways to change Kari's shortcomings, they strived to find resources that would allow Kari to reach her potential, no matter how small it was. It was critical for them. It was critical for Kari. At the time of her death, Kari was wheelchair dependent. She required constant care and feeding. She had little if any verbal communication skills. She attended a special-needs school and recognized family, friends, and teachers. She interacted with smiles and tears. Her quality of life was never in question. She participated to her fullest potential.

What was most remarkable was that her life was valued. Her parents never denied her existence. They never denied either, her condition. This was the only attitude they could realistically adopt. Some parents in their situation never find the commitment to achieve it. They become mired in emotions that distract from their ability to perhaps appreciate the fact that their child is alive and a part of them. They lose sight of the sincere effort of most clinicians to salvage the child's and family structure. Kari's parents were just as unique as Kari was. And that's why they worked so well together.

When Kari died, her mother quietly held her. Her bonus time had ended. In the pursuit of truth, I discovered my own shortcomings. I was—am—quick to judge and label. Perhaps because physicians must react quickly with little time to reflect on the potential shortcomings of any intervention. I began to realize that I would never be able to appreciate what my patients and their families feel unless I found new wisdom. Looking to Kari's mother, I found some.

"Kari didn't die because she had trisomy 18, did she? She died of chicken pox."

In her own way, she had made her point—subtle, yet concrete. Even by her death, Kari had refuted medical expectations.

A covenant relationship requires a willingness to listen

and learn. To recognize a person as a person. But with Kari I realized, finally, that the quality of life is simply the ability to give and receive love. No more, no less. I reflect on this as I continually transition to maturity as a physician. There's really no second chance in this business. But we can give more, care more, and love more. Perhaps that is, in the end, the best medicine.

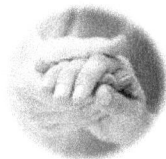

CHAPTER 22
THE DREAM

It had not been a particularly good week for the staff and patients in the pediatric critical care unit. Five deaths had destroyed us. Faced with our own inadequacies, we turned into malcontents, pessimists, and cynics. I set the tone for a crusade: save lives no matter the cost.

I sat in my office for a few minutes of quiet, laying my head on top of a book of medical history that I was reading. As I drifted into sleep, I heard a cough behind me. Turning, I saw a distinguished-looking gentleman, of genteel grace and culture, standing in the doorway. His large walrus mustache accentuated his balding head. A gold chain attached to one side of his vest swung across to the other side, lost in the vest pocket where his watch was housed. A high starched collar hid his neck.

"I have just finished walking through your ward and was delighted to see such wonderfully scientific tools at use," he said, entering my office and helping himself to my couch.

"Excuse me, sir, but you look very familiar," I queried, not sure what to expect next.

"What I look like is of no importance to you, young man. It is what I have to say that is. You've been having a rough time of it, haven't you?" he asked.

By now, I was sure I was dreaming. The gentleman looked as if he had come from another era. And yet, I knew him as if I had been around him for many years.

"Too many deaths," I sighed. "Sure, the ones we save are rewarding, but they are the easy ones. We're supposed to be able to save anybody and everybody."

"The trouble with you," he grumbled, "is that you're trying to practice medicine by rigid rules. You can't seek the answer to every diagnostic problem by a chemical reaction. You can't treat your patients by rule of thumb."

Who was this man? How dare he come in here and tell me how to practice medicine. If in fact he was a doctor, he was better suited for prescribing leeches or nondescript tonics.

"Curing of disease is not a realistic goal in your fancy ward. You are expected to reverse physiologic abnormalities and to buy time. I wish I could have been able to do that in my days. If your therapy works, then the body mounts its own attack," he continued.

Neither of us spoke for some time.

"Sometimes God just wants to make sure He's got your

attention. Medicine arose out of primal sympathy of man with man, out of the desire to help those in sorrow, need, and sickness. Nothing more, nothing less," he said, leaning forward, preparing to leave.

My beeper went off. I looked down to see myself raising my head off my arms to silence it. A vague dream had taken place. I looked to the couch. Stacks of paper lay where he had sat. I turned and looked at the book I was reading. William Osler, a mentor, had reached out.

My dream had reminded me, once again, that I had missed the purpose of medicine completely. People die. There is not much to say at such times, but much that needs to be said, ineffectual as it may be. It occurred to me, once again, that after all was said and done, there must be an absolute limit to intensive care if I am to use it wisely.

I walked back to the unit, pulled up a chair next to a child's bed, and spent the rest of the night sitting there, doing nothing more than holding her hand until she died.

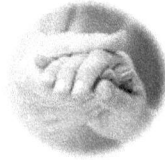

CHAPTER 23
HOPE, DIGNITY, AND RESPECT

I t's not always easy, though, these covenant relationships. It requires a commitment on your part, a responsibility to give your best to everyone, a willingness to find grace. Let me explain.

I am reminded of this again and again as I meet someone I have known for ten years. He's not a patient, but has come to be a friend. We met on the beach after I watched him for a few days, talking to some unknown person out there in the ocean, waving his hands and bowing. He spent days alone, lying on a dirty blanket, always in the same place right at the edge of the sand where it met with the high tide. He was the epitome of that type of person no one wants to claim. No one would sit next to him even when the beach was crowded. He wore the same clothes day in and day out, long hair matted, dirty fingernails, and drinking from a bottle in a paper bag. I was intrigued by his actions and embarrassed by the actions of others and myself: avoidance and distrust.

In the early evening, he would stand at the edge of the water, look west, and lift his hat and bow—to nobody. He would raise his hands, wave, and make the shape of a heart in the air, and I could hear him say, "I love you" over and over again. He would stay there and do this until the sun went down behind the horizon, and with his head hung low, shuffle up the beach and disappear for the night. I was determined to find out who he was and to whom he was talking to.

Approaching him on the beach late one afternoon, I introduced myself, and asked if he would like some company. Without any hesitation, he said yes. I sat down on a dirty blanket as the eyes of those around us all came into focus watching as a clean and well-groomed person sat close to a long-haired, dirty vagrant. For ten years, we met and talked for hours almost every day of my time on the beach each summer. Hugh is sixty-four years old, has two master's degrees, taught poetry in college, and lived *la vida loca* high on LSD from the time he was twenty until he crashed at the age of forty. He has been homeless off and on (more on than off) ever since. His mind is burned with LSD, flashbacks are frequent, but during his lucid times, he is smart, gentle, and humble.

Those times became fewer and fewer, and the last time I saw him, it was obvious that he was getting worse; he couldn't remember where he taught, went to college, or when we saw each other last. He slept in a park off the beach. I took him to one of our favorite places, Prince of Peace Abbey. We attended mass, prayed and talked for several hours, looking at the ocean from atop a hill where the abbey is. I listened as he moved from one subject to the next, sometimes making sense, most of the time not. We talked about Jo. She is the person he talks to, who he sees on the ocean in the evening—his love, his life. He says she lives on a sailboat and stays in the marina near the beach. I've checked. She doesn't exist. I've told him so, only to see his eyes water up and he becomes quiet, and he goes on talking about her as if he didn't hear me. I didn't bring it up anymore.

When I dropped him off at the park, I hugged him, held his hands as we prayed, and felt comfortable being with him despite what he was: a homeless, wasted, lonely man. I have grown to love him for who he is: a brother who seeks only that to which he is entitled to—dignity and personhood. He is not my patient. I don't have a duty to try to "save" him. But he has taught me something priceless. He is no different than the rest of us. We look to others for love and support, and welcome the warm embrace of those we love, the softness of a touch, the smell, the feel, the words, and the look they give us with their eyes. Hugh looks to Jo for all of that as well, raising his hat and waving his hands, making the shape of a heart with his hands to someone he loves out there in the ocean, wanting to feel her warmth. He believes in her. A fool's errand. But a sweet, gentle fool who lives a life as a consequence of what he did to himself in the past. I look past that and see in him the "forgotten children" who I care for in underprivileged countries. The innocent, abandoned, lonely, and forgotten children. I think of Hugh often as waves of sick and dying children cross my path daily. He gives me strength to keep moving forward, keep loving these children I care for with a soft touch, a warm hand.

Christ loves us unconditionally. A covenant relationship has that feel to it. It doesn't matter what the person looks like, smells like, and feels like. As doctors, we have elected to work with people—humans—to help heal their bodies. Bodies, as you all well know, are sometimes unpleasant. But that is why our calling is so precious. We have chosen that path, hopefully on purpose, and we must take on our calling with humility in our hearts and with grace, always ready to give and serve.

And that paper bag with the bottle in it? It was just water.

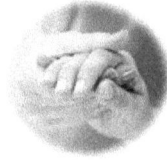

CHAPTER 24
MR. MORGAN

I've learned that the only difference between those who "have" and those who "have not" is what we decide to give or not give them. It's not about having or not having money, or access to medical technology, medicines, or even food or water. It's having or not having someone who cares enough to be by your side regardless. It's the ability to look beyond the grotesque. Yes, the grotesque. Physical and mental. The disfigured patient, the mentally unstable patient, the open wounds, the smells, the dying, and the hatred that hurting and ill patients exude when they have no one to be there with them. This "covenant," this relationship of trust, integrity, of being a servant, is that which gives those who have nothing, "something." A hand, a touch, love, compassion, and empathy. It takes courage to do that. It takes sacrifice to be the "good physician." The simple act of being present when present is what makes the difference when it comes to a relationship. I didn't learn this all overnight. In fact, I learned it from my patients, one at a time.

I was a second-year medical student. It was a Wednesday afternoon around 1:00 p.m. I remember the day vividly because Mr. Morgan was going to be my very first patient. I had my new white coat on with my nametag, a stethoscope, a reflex hammer, a penlight stuffed in my pocket, and a clipboard.

"Mr. Morgan, my name is David Beyda and I am a second-year medical student. I'd like your permission to ask you a few questions and to exam you."

"Come on in, Doctor," he said.

"I'm not a doctor, Mr. Morgan. I'm a second-year medical student."

Mr. Morgan had a cherubic face, soft blue eyes, wisps of white hair that lay in all directions begging to be combed, and a smile that invited anyone to smile back. He was frail but full spirited, with an enthusiasm that encouraged all those who came to know him to be the same.

"Come on in, Doctor. You've got a white coat on, don't you? Sit down and let's talk."

I pulled up a chair and placed it close to the right side of his bed, facing him.

"Come closer."

So I scooted up a little.

"Closer."

When I sat, he reached out to shake my hand. I could feel his transparent skin, his fingers curled and stiff with disease. And yet, his grip was strong, warm, and somehow comforting to this scared second-year medical student. He held on for a very long time. And I realized that the handshake had gone from simply that to a silent covenant.

As he held my hand, he began to tell me stories of his days as a patient, being chronically ill with liver cancer (he gave me his diagnosis, thank you very much), and how many doctors he had met along the way wearing white coats. I listened to him for a good while, as he told me all about those who were and who were not what he called "doctors."

He spoke of what I thought I already knew: kindness, compassion, empathy, and caring. I realized that the white coat I was wearing means something special, significant, important, and comforting to those who see us wearing it. I also got my first inkling that those who wear it don't necessarily embrace the same meaning.

When it finally came for me to do my history and physical, hours had gone by. For many days following, I returned and listened some more.

A few weeks later, I knocked on Mr. Morgan's door. He had been moved to an obscure area of the ward, a small isolated room distant from the nurse's station, distant from those to whom he had entrusted his care. I softly entered as his eyes were closed, and he looked like he was resting. I pulled up my chair to the usual place, took his hand, and held it like we had done many times before in the last few weeks, and waited. I waited to hear the stories, the encouragement, the critiques—no different, I realized, than I would hear from a parent. I listened. And all I heard was the soft, faint irregular breaths that he took as he moved on his journey towards a peaceful death. I listened, and then heard no more. Without any sense of shame or awkwardness, I kissed his forehead and simply said, "Thank you, Mr. Morgan," then walked out to let someone know that he had passed.

I regret not writing down all that Mr. Morgan had shared with me, but on rare occasions, a memory or two surfaces, bringing with them a smile and sense of gratitude for what he had shared with me. More important though, I remember the first gesture he made towards me—he wanted to hold my hand, and by him to doing so, I let myself be open to him as a human being, someone with feelings and needs beyond what mere medicine could give him. It took me a long time to really fully understand the gift Mr. Morgan gave me.

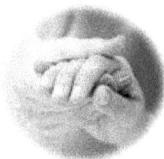

CHAPTER 25
CURE OR CARE

Sometimes, something will happen that leaves such an indelible mark on one's conscience that one is reminded of it frequently. Such a thing happened to me just recently—and I am constantly reminded of it. It was so stark I had hoped that over time, the footsteps of the memory would fade and I would no longer have to hear them. They have not. The footsteps keep marching.

In the late afternoon, two unrelated patients were admitted almost simultaneously. Both patients were critical—one child a submersion injury, the other a trauma. Both sustained significant neurological injury, and if they survived, both would be severely impaired. The parents of each child were as different from each other as the children themselves. Cultures and education aside, they had strikingly different expectations and needs. Nothing new so far—that happens weekly if not daily in my unit. What was so remarkably different was how they accepted the tragic event in their lives. And it is this difference that struck at the very heart of my conscience. At first, I fell into my usual mode. I began directing their lives, looking only one way. It was a very out-of-focus way because I began rushing to judgment.

One parent felt that his son could not, should not, be allowed to live a life suffering by being significantly disabled. The other parent felt that his son was worthy of life no matter his disability. They both were full of unconditional tender love for their child. I was to find myself in great conflict with one set of parents. The conflict centered on what I thought was humane, and what I thought was the right thing to do. It was not about success, and it starkly made me face up to what I felt success was. For success, as I argued above, is defined as "curing," but in neither case was "cure" possible. But what happened was, I was faced with my ideas about the advance of science and its power.

We invented science, and with its advance we create moral dilemmas that science by itself cannot resolve. Abraham Flexner in 1925 described the ideal physician as an educated person in whom science and humanity are necessarily and indissolubly united. The basis of humanity stems from the simple notion of humanism. Humanism, loosely defined, is simply a mere slogan that raises expectations that are doomed to collapse. For me, humanism is the unselfish compassion for another human being. I assume life is valued unless there is evidence to show that it is not. This sense of compassion is in all of us who are in medicine. We have somehow become uncomfortable with it, or at least cynical in its use.

It drives us to look often for what we think is right and not necessarily what is demanded. It sits right at the heart of the "healing" versus "curing" debate. Many opportunities to heal are still lost as physicians choose to restrict their gaze to the technical aspects of cure. We can overcome this by simply caring. However, to care for someone where there is no reciprocation can lead to exhaustion and depletion. Caring should occur simply, spontaneously, and without effort. Today, caring is buried because of strained relationships. Medicine should be a relationship of persons. The ideal physician is perhaps one who is fully engaged in meaningful relationships with his patients—a task we are finding increasingly hard to do. And when it comes to communication, it is not necessarily what we say, but how we say it.

Like it or not, we are obsessed with two self-serving agendas: what we want and how do we get it. The irony of this is that when we do get it, it is not needed anymore, or if it is truly a want it is never enough. In medicine this seems to hold true as well. To pursue these two agendas goes against the very ethic inherent to medicine. We have fallen victim to ourselves. Four questions need to be asked concerning any human who is ill: what is wrong, what will happen, what can be done, and what should be done? These four questions need to be answered by both physician and patient. It cannot be one-sided.

I have had to learn the value of these questions the hard way. And I have learned to ask more: whose point of view are we taking when we deal with our patients? To look at the case from our point of view places personal values on somebody else. To look at the case from the patient's point of view is a more difficult task. Physicians should be morally mature people who have chosen certain values consciously. We are identified by the values we espouse, and even more so by the values we evidence in our daily decisions and activities. It is not necessarily what we should do, but how we do it and when. So the question really becomes, as a result of something we do, are our patients better off?

For the two sets of parents with severely impaired children, my personal values should have held little weight in what they wanted for their children. What was important for them was the type of relationship they had with their child. How I ensured that relationship was of paramount importance to them. I learned very quickly that sick persons are not consumers of our product, or clients—contrary to what the current medical culture would like us to believe. They are patients: persons suffering, bearing an illness, in need of relief which we are called on to provide as best we can. These two children deserved as much, and I faltered in giving it to them because of my insistence on what I thought was right rather than doing what was best.

You, perhaps, are comfortable with who you are and what you want. I certainly thought I was. The search for answers to the questions posed continues. It is for me a task of humility and testimony, both of which are difficult roads for me to travel.

The issues of how far do we push technology are not always easy. There are no clear answers sometimes. Fortunately, for the most part, most cases are straightforward, the questions easily answered. In the end, however, our own minds must be satisfied and that is the toughest taskmaster.

Curing disease is not always a realistic goal of an intensive care unit. We can certainly reverse acute physiologic abnormalities and buy some time. If our therapy works, then the body mounts its own attack and the patient may live. We can also prolong the dying process. But there is a limit to technology. There is a point where we must recognize when we're moving away from trying to care for our patient to being that god in a white coat and working to cure our patients—even when no cure is possible. We must acknowledge an absolute limit to intensive care if we are to use it wisely. I strive to achieve this limit, but at times I am unsuccessful.

It's a complex issue, the one I raised above. Where do we draw the line between "cure" and "care"?

The simple truth is, most health-insurance companies are demanding more for their dollars and paying out less. That model demands that physicians need to see more patients in less time, with restrictions that take away from the doctor's ability to really get to know and establish a relationship with the patient. Instead, both the doctor and the patient enroll in health-insurance plans and they are assigned a patient and a doctor respectively. This is far from the old days of when physicians and patients came together based on shared values, small-town cultures, covenant relationships that went beyond just that within a family.

So that, again, begs the question. Is the physician doing what he should be doing or what he wants to be doing?

Behavior directs care, and it is culture driven. It seems that some physicians have a tendency to follow a norm of doing what they want on a personalized or directed level rather than on the level of the patient's best interests. In other words, are physicians doing what is right and not necessarily what is demanded of them? When we look at the current issue of managed care, the "gatekeeper," a physician who directs patient medical care from a distance, often succumbs to administrative pressures to contain costs. I often find that these "gatekeepers" can be classified as two types: the "gate slammers" and the "gate openers." The "gate slammers" are fearful of the managed care's administrative power and therefore follow to the letter the dictum of cost containment, often neglecting the best interest of the patient. The "gate openers" are interested in recovery of the patient and will do their best to find the right solution for the patient's welfare. They encourage and mobilize the patient to heal.

The gate slammer is more interested in the contract between the patient and the doctor. The patient comes to the doctor through his insurance company. The patient is a "client"; it is a business relationship whereby the patient contracts with that particular doctor to get the best medical advice to fix his problem. The doctor takes no time to find out who that person is.

I cite this example again to show what I mean. A patient is ushered into your examining room. He's got abdominal pain. He said, "I get it every day. It's associated with meals. If I drink milk it's okay." Sounds like an ulcer, so you give him an antacid. He comes back two weeks later because he still has pain. In other words, he still didn't get "fixed"—and that's the key; he's not fixed so he thinks you're a lousy physician. It is the downside of the contract relationship. The patient is paying, often a premium price, for a service so he expects positive results. If it doesn't happen, he grumbles about the state of health care these days, or worst case, he sues.

Now here's the catch. It's all covered under the insurance. You did exactly what managed care dictated you do. But how cost effective was the treatment?

The "gate openers" would allow physicians to do things a little different. They would be encouraged to ask the patient, "Mr. Jones, tell me about the pain." He does. But before I think "ulcer" and write the prescription, I ask, "What's your normal day like?"

He starts telling you, "I'm a plumber, and things haven't been good this year." With a little more prodding you find out he doesn't need an antacid; he needs someone to help him get over the anxiety. Sure, the antacid might help, but if he's in your office again in two weeks, you're back to square one. The same discussion can be had with the villager in Africa, a garbage collector in Egypt, or a beggar in a slum in India. The "who" before the "what."

A question physicians need to constantly ask themselves is, "As a result of something I did, are my patients better off?" Unfortunately the question most posed by doctors these days is, "Did I do everything humanly possible to cure my patient and if I lost them, well, I did everything possible." The two questions are fundamentally different, and one is more patient centered, while the other is more concerned with making sure the doctor thinks he or she is right.

None of us should be in the game of seeing who can be more right about someone's healthcare. Rather, we should be concerned about finding a way to get the patient back to good health—or letting them die peacefully, with dignity and grace.

Another issue fuels the fire. Patient autonomy has come to the fore. With the increase in public knowledge and sophistication, and necessitated by the overwhelming choices offered by technological advances, patients have become more aggressive in demanding a more active part in the decision-making process. They demand more, but more of what?

Years ago patients could be sure that their personal physician was truly their advocate and was always acting in their best interests—as healer when possible but always as a caring companion. Such assurance brought with it the confidence there was a trusting role doctors used to play in their patients' lives.

⌒∞⌒

"Hanging of Crepe" is a technique of communication used by some physicians, a technique that is described in the medical literature. The patient must be critically ill, but it can work in most any situation. The strategy is to paint the most pessimistic picture, thereby ensuring a "no-lose" situation: nature kills; the physician saves if he can. Hanging of crepe is not new. An anonymous physician of the School of Solerno in the 12th century stated: "when examining the urine you should observe its color, substance, quantity, and content; after which you may promise the patient that with the help of God you will cure him. As you go away, however, you should say to his servants that he is in a very bad way, because if he recovers you will receive great credit and praise and if he dies, they will remember that you despaired of his health from the beginning." (*Anonymi salernitani De adventu medici ad aegrotum*, in Salvaroe de Renzi, *Collectio Salernitana*, Napopli, Filiatre-Sebezio, 1852-1859, 5 Vols. II, pp 74-75.) Hanging of the crepe is ethically unjust and against the moral standing of honesty. It's something we do sometimes do to ensure we win either way.

I have found that contrary to what the current lay

healthcare gurus are projecting, our patients really want more than a scientist—they want the healer who is also caring. Patients want the doctor to be a friend and confidant as well as a competent, scientifically up-to-date physician. There are times, however, when I've come across a patient or a family who clearly wants a "scientist" to be the physician in charge and dispense with the caring and compassion and look solely to the "cure." That at times comes with "expectations" that are sometimes far from realistic and sets everyone up for failure.

So when did "caring" get buried by "curing"?

The physician's task is not to only cure an illness, but to care for patients. One needs to act rightly at the right time for the right reasons in the right manner. The "process" of care rather than the goal of care seems to be a primary intent of some clincians. We need to consider the intent versus the motive. The fact of the matter is that we don't care, we don't have time to care, we don't know how to care, and patients sometimes don't want caring.

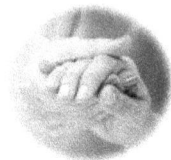

CHAPTER 26
CARING OR CURING—IT IS UP TO US TO DECIDE

Health care has definitely put a certain spin on what we consider good health "care." But what it really comes down to, for both the patient and the doctor, is this: is your priority curing or caring? We need to address the issues of care as they relate to cure first. Do patients receive the care they need? Do patients need the care they receive? In other words, as a result of something physicians do, are their patients better off? Today, patients are expected to recover. When they don't, then the assumption is that someone is at fault. Caring is skewed as a result.

I believe that there is a big difference between "caring about," "to take care of," and "to care for." Each demonstrates a different type of caring, and one could argue that each type of caring is unique. How would you demonstrate each? Would it be related to time? Would it be related to actions? Would it be a form of charity?

What I have found over the years in my pediatric

intensive-care unit is **how** one does what one does is as important as **what** one does. When we act responsibly, our attitude is such that we begin to care, and with that caring comes compassion. We must become aware of our habits. What specific habits do you bring to the bedside? And why? The answers are hard to come by sometimes, aren't they?

It's interesting to see who we are on the first day of being a physician, and who we have become by the last day. The changes are dramatic—in our emotions, our expectations, our outlook, and our understanding of life. We come with an attitude of "giving" and leave with a gratitude of "receiving." We always leave with more than we came with...I think you know what I mean. Our expectations are somewhat skewed until we realize that it is not about "what," but about "who." The greatest tool we bring to the patients we'll see in our practices of medicine is ourselves.

I ask the question over and over again: for what purpose are we here? And after some thought, it becomes clearer. To serve those who have nothing, who in some of the countries I've traveled to, out of desperation, will give up their own children to ensure their children will have a better life. To serve those who come to us for help and who have no choice but to trust us. To realize our own shortcomings and our inadequacies. But above all to give those who are hurting a chance to have their dignity and to be recognized as persons embraced for who they are. It makes me wonder why it is sometimes so hard to do. If you have embraced the "covenant" with your patient, then it isn't hard. I hope that it's not that hard tomorrow, or the day after, or the day after that.

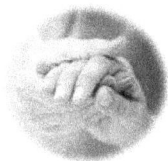

CHAPTER 27
SECOND-GUESSING

One of the best things about age, it is said, is that it can bring with it a certain perspective. Many years of practicing critical care medicine has left me wondering how come technology has been unable to keep up with wisdom.

Osler taught that medicine arose out of primal sympathy of man with man, out of the desire to help those in sorrow, need, and sickness. Critical care medicine has evolved as a discipline that implies to both lay people and health professionals alike, the certainty of life. It's all in the mystique, I suppose, but the mystique of saving lives is based only on the reality that technology can, in fact, keep almost anybody "alive."

When I saw Gloria for the last time a few weeks ago, her mind was fully occupied with the immediate, brief future. Aplastic anemia had thrown down the gauntlet. She lived with us for two months. We rallied 'round Gloria and won many small battles, calling on conventional resources and finally on some unconventional ones.

Her mother was a lady of gentle grace, unable at times to communicate because of a language barrier. She always refused to discuss the irreversibility of Gloria's illness. She never denied it. She just refused to accept it. We were as guilty of this as she was.

We repeatedly asked Gloria's mother for a DNR. She always said no. It occurred to me later that after all was said and done, we really shouldn't have offered CPR as a choice. Offering CPR represented bad faith. Doing so implied potential benefit when there was none. Must we use CPR? Must we always seek permission to not resuscitate? Was there an obligation to keep this patient alive?

Gloria was extubated several days before she died. She was coherent and made a strong statement for wanting to go home before she died. Because critical care medicine had, up to this point, been so successful in beating the odds, it was decided to continue with our aggressive approach. Early one morning she had a massive bleed into her brain and she died a few hours later. At first I was stunned; I remembered how we were able to pull her through so many times before. And then I started to get angry. Saving Gloria's life was nothing other than a vague dream and pleasant fantasy. We had, perhaps, lost the purpose of practicing medicine.

I have never come up with anything that might generously be called a stroke of genius. I sometimes, however, realize my shortcomings. Technology, no questions asked, has ensured that many, many children are alive today. Wisdom, on the other hand, has ensured that we need to keep things in perspective. Curing of disease is not always a realistic goal of an intensive care unit. We can certainly reverse acute physiologic abnormalities and buy some time. If our therapy works, then the body mounts its own attack. We can also prolong the dying process. We must acknowledge an absolute limit to intensive care if we are to use it wisely. I strive to achieve this limit but at times I am unsuccessful. Granted, Gloria's is a most odious example. For the most part, the cases are straightforward, the questions easily answered. In the end, however, our own minds must be satisfied, and that is the toughest taskmaster.

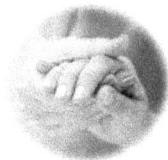

CHAPTER 28
WE ARE WHO WE ARE

A while back I had an experience that brought back memories of times gone past, when I was a "god in a white coat." A sick child was urgently admitted to the unit from the emergency department with little that I could do to change the course of the disease. I could see the fulminant infection spreading quickly through his little body, his organs failing, and the alarms chirping their incessant warning that all was to collapse even if I did try to do something. I had learned long ago that just because we can do something, there are many reasons why we shouldn't. We yield to the temptation of wanting to cure at the consequence of invoking needless suffering and pain. It doesn't mean that there are not times when we should pursue all heroic measures. Critical care is all about that, and more often than not we win the battle. But, there is a limit to what we should put our patients through. We need to think of the consequences of what we do to our patients. It was clear that the end was near for this child, and even if I could do something "to" that little child, it would not yield anything "for" that child. The best I could do and the most important thing I could and should do, was to ensure that the child didn't suffer, feel any pain, and above all have the child's dignity respected. I went to his mother and held her for a moment as she wept. We hadn't even been introduced to each other yet. I was meeting her and her son for the first time. I asked if she had a faith she turned to in difficult times. She said she was a Christian. This struck a chord in me, remembering the mother from Flagstaff. This time, I simply said, "pray with me." As we prayed, the little boy died, as God had decided. Not me. The mother cried and held her little boy, and softly whispered, "He is yours, God." What a difference when we have a God in whom we believe and trust. What a difference He has made in my life.

∞

As I watch the team in the PICU doing what they do best, I smile. A young baby, illness untreatable, comes off life support. There is an intense love for this little being, the unquestioning respect for the dignity of the child, and the selfless acts of genuine caring for that child. It is all done without prompting or protocol. It just happens. As I watch and listen, there is silence and I smile. There was no need for words, just actions. Everybody got it. Shared values and commitment. A family of dedicated unpretentious people, doing what comes from the gifts that they have been given. When we do what we believe in, serving others in need, unselfishly and together, the sad times hurt less and the joyous times are more joyous.

When you look in the mirror, what do you see? *Whom do*

you see? The reflection shows the "what" but not the "who"—the person inside. I hope my words have caused you to reflect more on the "who" instead of the "what."

For what it's worth, the more you show of who you are, the better off you are. And what I have learned in my years of practicing medicine, here in one of the most privileged nations on earth and in some places that can only be described as hell, is that the highest expectations should come from the person you're looking at in the mirror: the "who."

Over the past years I have come to realize that patients, in the end, really want to know that someone will look after them. They want reassurance. They want to know that we are focused on their well being. And so I ask again, are our patients better off because of what we do "to" them, or are our patients better off because of what we do "for" them?

∽∞∾

I remember the first time that I helped with the delivery of the baby, seeing a beating heart in surgery, my first death, my first mistake, the first time I had to tell the truth to a patient, the first time I made a brilliant diagnosis, and the first time I missed the diagnosis, the first time a patient came back to tell me thank you, and the first time a patient told me that they hated me. There are many more first times and we all go through them. I remember holding the hand of a patient who could not respond because they were heavily sedated on life-support, and how vulnerable I felt and how humbling it was to know that all I could offer was comfort and yet how privileged it was to do so.

Will our relationship with our patients be a contract or covenant? And will it be sincere or superficial? Patients trust their physicians because they have no choice but to trust them. All of this impacts other people every day of our lives, for better or worse, and sometimes we're ignorant of what we've left behind.

Practicing medicine is a learning task from our first patient to our last night on call, and it's been said that knowledge is proud that he has learned so much and wisdom is humble that he knows no more. How true that is. For me it is also something else. Humility. The grace of humility is a precious gift. The judgment of others doesn't matter because we know what we've done. So for me I remember my own imperfections, and when I do the faults of others seem less grievous. I am not a god in a white coat. I am simply a silent servant practicing with my heart as well as my head, helping those who are vulnerable and sick as they reach out their hand for help. A *covenant* relationship.

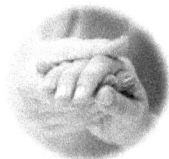

CHAPTER 29
HOW IT CAME TO BE

It seems like coincidence finds its way into our lives when we least expect it. Some say that a coincidence is simply God's way of tapping us on the shoulder. It happened all the same, and for me, God tapped me on the shoulder. Rather sharply.

Soon after I found myself playing a "god in a white coat," I was invited to be a Visiting Scholar and Visiting Fellow at the Center for Clinical Ethics and the Rose Kennedy Institute of Ethics at Georgetown. For several years I traveled back and forth from my home to Washington DC every week, basking in the teachings of great scholars in ethics and medicine. Dr. Edmund Pellegrino was a mentor to me like no other. A world-renowned Christian ethicist, he taught me all about virtue and what he meant by always being there for the "patient's good." I was far from being faith based, but enjoyed the discussions, the debates, and yes, the challenges he posed of me both from a personal perspective and a professional one. He grounded me from a moral and ethical perspective as it related to patient care: the patient first always. After several years of traveling to Washington DC weekly, I began to lose focus on my purpose and priorities. One Sunday I was attending church because of Charlcye, my wife, and the boys. Rev. Stanley was the pastor of the church, and during the many years that I knew him we spoke many times about my weak faith, where I was in my own spiritual growth, my exposure to Christ and what that meant to me. And because of that, I sensed that he had a genuine concern for my spiritual growth. Remember, I took care of his granddaughter many years before, and so we had a special relationship. On a particular Sunday morning, he mentioned to me that there was going to be a men's retreat called a "Walk to Emmaus" in which he was going to be the spiritual leader. This retreat was well attended and there was a two-year waiting list to get a spot. He suggested that I call the next day to get myself on the list for the next available spot. He thought it would help me through whatever my issues were with faith. The fact was, however, that the retreat was for Christian men, of which I wasn't. I called the next morning. The lady who answered listened to my request to be put on a waiting list. She said she was expecting my call. There had been a cancellation just a few minutes earlier, and she was putting me on the list for this retreat that Rev. Stanley was going to be the spiritual leader on. Two weeks later, with Rev. Stanley, I accepted Christ. Circumstances, coincidences, God's hand—who knows? It's all about faith.

My life changed after that. Within 24 hours, I was a new me. My practice of medicine changed, I started praying with patients, becoming humble, and becoming a gentler, selfless person. In 1996, my faith was born; I shed my ego and began to have a covenant relationship with my patients.

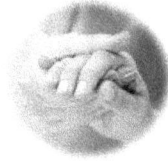

CHAPTER 30
SELF-REFLECTION

This is a whole new life, this covenant-versus-contract relationship in medicine. It is not a momentary act, practice, common routine, or schedule. It is a commitment and a reverence to who we are as physicians and our responsibilities to our patients not to live our lives as gods in white coats but as silent servants. What is important is what we do with our lives and who and what we become and where we go. I was a do-gooder motivated by my own need to be needed or to make a notable difference and found that instead of true compassion and commitment to meet human needs, it was all about me. I am cautious, however. Things change, so they say, but in reality only I have changed. Everything will be the same if I am not truly committed to who I am. People may or may not be interested in what I do or say, and at times I have felt discouraged and empty. It is easy to bask in a new life only to find old habits and routines coming back. I found that there are two dangers in my life. Believing that I was someone special, and now believing that I am still someone special and different. I have recognized that there are priorities, and recognize that there is a reality and that I am not necessarily better but simply one who feels more comfortable with who I am and who I should be. I'm more comfortable with seeking tolerance and mutual understanding. I'm willing to put myself in someone else's shoes and to take the focus off myself and imagine what it's like to be in someone else's predicament and simultaneously feel love for that person. I realize that everyone is different and no one has the same capabilities as the next, and that by showing grace, by understanding, a foundation for covenant relationships is formed. I make the best use of what is in my power and I take the rest as it happens. I believe that I am part of a created order and God is active in sustaining this creation, and this God is closely accessible to me and to everyone and we participate by believing in Him.

To say that I have a singular vision of what it means to be a physician is very far from the truth. All I have is exposure to a whole lot of experience and events, each of which brings with it a unique message and point. It is from these encounters and events that I write, giving a simple perspective as to what it means to me and how I see it affecting those who are involved. Practicing pediatric critical care medicine, caring for children who are dying or close to it, has given me an opportunity to question my own strengths and weaknesses, my own morality, and my own purpose. I have learned to look at what is important, to ask why I do this work and to what end. It is never easy to look or see what is in front of us, especially when it is distasteful. There are times when medicine is distasteful. There are many more times when medicine is just fine. To differentiate between the two seems simple enough for those who are discerning and specific. For those who are at times confused, the difference is difficult to see. And that is where faith comes in.

I have found that what we do is not as important as who we are. We are science centered and art poor. Medicine as a science is on a fast track. It is curing patients with all the tools we have available to us. We have an enormous amount of research and technology to assist us in our quest to heal people. We order tests and use expensive drugs to heal. We do all of that well, and many are saved because of it. We have insurance companies who broker our relationships with our patients. Physicians use insurance companies as brokers to find patients. Patients use insurance companies as brokers to find physicians. We are advancing logarithmically, moving into new territory daily, finding ways to make a diagnosis with technology, make new medicines, and decreasing mortality as a result. Science can be a world of constants, rules, and processes that can always be counted on. Science is also at times cold, unfeeling, and exceedingly inhuman. Science is enriching for the mind but not always so enriching for the soul. However, medicine is also an art, the caring side of medicine, and it is falling quickly into an abyss where it may possibly lay unnoticed simply because nobody will look for it or even want it.

I'd like us to think about what this *covenant relationship* in medicine is. If you're a patient, do you judge your doctor on how well he or she performs or how much they care about you as a person? I have found over the years that patients want to know that someone will look after them, and they want reassurance that you are focused on their well-being. It's easy to take "care of" someone, but it is more difficult and more burdensome at times to "care about" or to "care for" someone. Are our patients better off because of *what we do "to" them*, or are they better off because of *what we do "for" them*? Doing something "to" someone is relatively easy to do. It is a contract. It has measurable results. It is procedural in nature and may or may not have any benefit. But when we think about doing something "for" someone, it implies a commitment and inherent willingness to have a relationship with someone. With that come responsibilities and commitment, and that is the *covenant* of which I speak.

Here is a challenge: hold the hand of a patient who can't respond either because they are heavily sedated or are unconscious, and feel how vulnerable we are as physicians, how humbling it is knowing that all we can offer sometimes is comfort. I hope it brings home how privileged it is to be able to do so. It is that privilege that establishes the covenant with another person. The willingness to give of oneself, to sacrifice, to look beyond the grotesque and feel comfortable with just who you are and who the patient is; no pretense, no fanfare, no expectations—nothing other than a relationship based on trust, honesty, and integrity.

There are many physicians who practice good covenant

medicine. They know the value of building trust with their patients, finding out who they are and how they can best help them. If you're reading this, I hope that you find it to be an acknowledgment. But as I train new residents and medical students, I can't help but think of the irony of the white coat that is worn. Wearing the white coat takes on the image of a "god in a white coat." We've earned those white coats. But it takes time to learn what it means to be a physician. We put on the white coat with confidence and pride, but we need to wear it with humility.

I say again that the greatest task we face as physicians is to decide who we are and what our relationship with our patients is going to be. Will it be a *contract* or *covenant*? The most powerful tool that a physician can bring to the bedside is himself. Patients trust their physicians because they have no choice but to trust them. All of us impact other people every day of our lives for better or for worse; sometimes, though, we are ignorant of what we leave behind. A lot has changed in my practice of medicine. It took faith, commitment, humility, and an understanding of what it means to be something greater than myself. As we decide "who" we are in relationship to our patients, we begin to understand that it is not the "what" but the "who" that is most important. The patient, not always the disease. The person, not always the body. We should strive to focus on the dignity of the person, and in doing so, we will find ourselves caring enough to want to cure.

And remember baby Nicole? A few months ago, my wife and I attended her wedding. Nicole graduated from college *summa cum laude* and she is now a graduate student—smart, beautiful, and without any limitations from her time as a sick baby. A baby I took off life support to allow her to die. It's all about faith. Covenant medicine. Being present when present. What a wonderful way to practice medicine.